The Menopause

Dr Sarah Brewer MA, MB, BChir

THE MENOPAUSE

Thorsons
An Imprint of HarperCollins*Publishers*

Thorsons
An Imprint of HarperCollins*Publishers*
77–85 Fulham Palace Road,
Hammersmith, London W6 8JB
1160 Battery Street,
San Francisco, California 94111–1213
Published by Thorsons 1997

10 9 8 7 6 5 4 3 2 1

A catalogue record for this book
is available from the British Library

ISBN 0 7225 3389 6

Printed and bound in Great Britain by
Caledonian International Book Manufacturing Ltd, Glasgow

To Richard and Saxon

CONTENTS

PREFACE: THE ESSENTIAL GUIDE SERIES

This series offers up-to-date, in-depth information on common health problems. These books contain detailed, medically accurate information in a user-friendly, easy to read style.

Each book covers:

- What the condition is
- How common it is
- Who is affected by it
- Normal body functions and how each condition affects them
- Symptoms
- Causes
- Risk factors
- How the condition is diagnosed – blood tests, investigations, etc.
- Other similar conditions that need to be ruled out
- The drugs used to treat it – including side-effects and who shouldn't take them
- Surgical treatments that can help
- Complementary treatments
- Self-help tips
- Dietary changes that may prove helpful
- Latest research findings
- Addresses of support groups and sources of further information

This invaluable series will answer all your questions and help you to make the best decisions regarding your own health care.

Chapter One

AN INTRODUCTION TO THE MENOPAUSE AND HRT

For many women, the menopause is a welcome time of life. It signals the end of the monthly menstrual cycle and marks the beginning of a new phase of life.

It is triggered once your ovaries run out of eggs and your levels of the female hormone, oestrogen, fall. This deprives the lining of your womb (endometrium) of its normal source of stimulation and your periods stop altogether. This may happen suddenly, or you may notice a gradual change in your usual menstrual cycle so that your periods become increasingly erratic and irregular.

The menopause is really a long-term process that may start at the age of 40 but is not actually finished until you reach the age of 50 or more. The menopause itself is said to date from your last actual period – but this can only be discovered with hindsight, after a woman of suitable age, with classic symptoms, has not had a period for at least a year. All the symptoms and period problems you may have noticed up until your periods stop – as well as afterwards – are more properly known as *perimenopausal* symptoms, as they occur *around* the time of your menopause.

For most women, their last natural period occurs between the ages of 45 and 55, with a UK average of 51 years. As a modern woman can expect to live well into her eighties, as much as 40 per cent of her active life may occur after her last period.

Many women find it a relief not to have to cope with irregular, heavy or painful bleeding each month, nor worry about unwanted pregnancy. Most will have finished raising their families by this time as well, so will have more time to spend enjoying themselves.

Your experience of the menopause will depend on your particular circumstances, lifestyle and how your body copes with falling levels of oestrogen. While 1 in 4 women sails through with few problems, 3 out of 4 suffer physical and emotional symptoms which can be debilitating. In particular, women who lead a demanding, stressful life seem more likely to suffer distressing symptoms. This is probably because their adrenal glands – which usually double the output of certain sex hormones to make up for the lower levels produced by the ovaries – are already working flat out at the menopause and do not have the reserves to produce increased amounts of hormones which can help to even out some of the fluctuations occurring around this time of life (*see page 26*).

Although it is easy to pigeon-hole the menopause as a deficiency disease, it is important to remember that it is a natural event. Your body is designed to stop making oestrogen and to adjust to the changes this brings. Even so, the last thing most women want to bother with are distressing menopausal symptoms and long-term health problems linked with lowered levels of oestrogen.

Women are now in the best possible position to enjoy their post-menopausal years. On the one hand, hormone replacement therapy (HRT) can free you from the burden of unwanted menopausal symptoms and has the potential to prolong your life by postponing the development of osteoporosis and coronary heart disease (CHD). On the other, women who are unable – or unwilling – to take artificial hormone treatment, can access a wide range of complementary therapies as well as making dietary and lifestyle changes to help them get through what can – but doesn't have to be – a difficult time of life.

HORMONE REPLACEMENT THERAPY

While HRT remains controversial, benefits are increasingly being discovered which outweigh the possible risks. HRT aims to give you back the natural levels of oestrogen which your ovaries are no longer making so that, overall, your body's exposure to hormones is usually less than if your ovaries were to continue working efficiently themselves. As a result, the risks and benefits of HRT are very different from those of, for example, the oral contraceptive pill, which is designed to cause artificially high hormone levels similar to those found during pregnancy.

Unfortunately, it is common for HRT to be tarred with the same brush as the oral contraceptive pill. In fact, some experts now feel that the only true contraindication to taking HRT is the presence of an active hormone-sensitive tumour such as breast cancer. Once this has been treated, however, new research shows that even women who have previously had breast cancer can safely take HRT in many cases.

The decision about whether or not to take HRT is a very personal one, which only you can make after a full discussion with your doctor and having weighed up the possible risks and benefits involved (for more information, *see Chapter 7*).

Chapter Two

MENSTRUATION AND THE MENOPAUSE

THE NORMAL MENSTRUAL CYCLE

In order to understand the changes that occur at the menopause – and why they happen – it is worth reviewing the normal female reproductive system. Your menstrual cycle is controlled by a group of chemical messengers known as sex hormones. These are made in three different parts of your body:

1. the pituitary gland in the base of the brain
2. the hypothalamus – a part of the brain just above the pituitary gland
3. your ovaries (female gonads).

The Pituitary Gland

The pituitary gland is a pea-sized structure which hangs down from the base of your brain on a short stalk. It is sometimes referred to as the master gland, as it is the most important of your endocrine (hormone-producing) glands. It releases several hormones, of which two help to regulate your menstrual cycle:

1. follicle stimulating hormone (FSH)
2. leutinizing hormone (LH)

These two hormones are together known as gonadotrophins as they stimulate your sex glands, or gonads (the testicles in males and the ovaries in females).

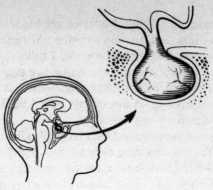

The pituitary gland

The Hypothalamus

The hypothalamus is the part of your brain situated directly above the pituitary gland. It produces several hormones, one of which, gonadotrophin releasing hormone – or GnRH for short – triggers the production of FSH and LH in the pituitary gland. GnRH is released in short bursts and, as a result, production of FSH and LH also occurs in short pulses throughout the day and night, rather than at a steady level.

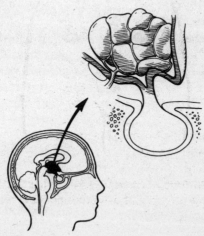

The hypothalamus

The Ovaries

The two female sex glands, or ovaries, are made up of two zones: an inner medulla and an outer cortex. At birth, a baby girl is born with ovaries that contain around 2 million immature eggs, known as oocytes. Some of these immature eggs slowly disintegrate and are reabsorbed during childhood – and throughout life – in a process known as atresia. By the time of puberty, only around half a million eggs remain.

Each oocyte is surrounded by a layer of cells to form an ovarian follicle. The surrounding cells are full of tiny granules rich in cholesterol which will be converted into the female sex hormones, oestrogen and progesterone, once the ovaries are activated at puberty.

Oestrogen produced by the ovaries after puberty travels back to both the hypothalamus and the pituitary gland to turn them down a bit and regulate the amount of GnRH, LH and FSH they produce. The ovaries also produce a hormone called inhibin, which travels back to the pituitary gland to reduce FSH production. These feedback mechanisms are clever ways of making sure the ovaries are not over-stimulated to produce too many eggs.

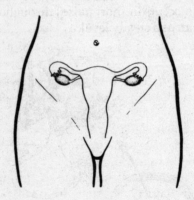

The ovaries

The Start of the Menstrual Cycle

The first period (menarche) normally occurs between the ages of 10 and 16, but occasionally occurs earlier or later than this. Puberty is triggered by an unknown signal that causes the hypothalamus to start producing pulses of GnRH. This hormone passes down to the pituitary gland and stimulates production of Follicle Stimulating Hormone (FSH) and Leutinizing Hormone (LH). These two hormones are secreted directly into the bloodstream and travel to the ovaries, where they act as the signal for fertile life to begin.

As its name suggests, FSH triggers the production and development of a number of ovarian follicles. On average, around 15 eggs start to ripen at the beginning of each cycle. As well as growing in size, these follicles secrete the female hormone, oestrogen, and blood levels of oestrogen start to rise. One follicle eventually outstrips the rest and for some reason is chosen to become 'follicle of the month'. It produces increasing amounts of oestrogen, which have a damping effect on the pituitary gland in the brain. As a result, blood levels of FSH fall slightly. When this happens, the other follicles stop growing and start to regress. Only the dominant follicle is mature enough to continue responding to the lower levels of FSH. This dominant follicle continues to grow while the others break down and disappear. FSH then continues to act on the layer of cells surrounding the egg in this follicle to stimulate increased production of oestrogen hormone.

There are two main peaks of oestrogen production – one just before ovulation from the dominant follicle, and another smaller one around a week later. As blood levels of oestrogen start to rise at the beginning of your menstrual cycle, the lining of the womb (endometrium) responds by starting to thicken up. Growth of the endometrium is rapid during the first two weeks of the menstrual cycle, which is known as the proliferative (or follicular) phase. By the time ovulation occurs, the endometrial lining is ready and waiting for the possible implantation of a fertilized egg.

As the dominant follicle matures, the egg inside becomes suspended on a hillock within a large, fluid-filled cavity which measures 2–3 cm across and bulges from the surface of the ovary.

Just before ovulation, the pituitary gland secretes a sudden flood of FSH and LH in what is known as the LH surge. This triggers ovulation around 9 hours later and the dominant follicle bursts, releasing its mature egg (ovum). Some women notice mid-cycle pain at around this time due to the pressure within the swollen egg follicle.

As a rule, only one egg is released each month. Contrary to popular belief, an egg is not released from each ovary on alternate months. There doesn't seem to be a standard; eggs are released from the two ovaries in an irregular and unpredictable pattern.

The Corpus Luteum

After ovulation, the empty ovarian follicle that has just released an egg collapses and fills with blood. The cells surrounding the follicle, which are rich in cholesterol granules, rapidly grow and divide until the clotted blood within the collapsed follicle is replaced with yellowish, fatty cells to form a yellow cyst – the corpus luteum.

For around 10 days after ovulation, the cyst swells until it is around 2 cm across. During this time it continues making oestrogen and also starts to secrete lots of another female hormone, progesterone. This is known as the luteal, or secretory phase of the menstrual cycle.

The Luteal Phase

Up until ovulation, the endometrium has been thickening up (proliferating) under the influence of oestrogen. As soon as ovulation occurs, the corpus luteum produces increasing amounts of progesterone which trigger changes in the endometrium. Blood vessels rapidly grow into the thickened womb lining so it becomes soft, spongy, vascular and boggy. Its glands start to secrete a clear, nourishing fluid – this part of the menstrual cycle is known as the secretory phase. The secretions are designed to provide a fertilized egg with vital nutrients both before and after it implants.

Maintaining Early Pregnancy

If pregnancy occurs, the implanted fertilized egg starts to produce a hormone known as human Chorionic Gonadotrophin (hCG).

This acts as a signal to the corpus luteum cyst in one of the ovaries to continue producing progesterone. Progesterone hormone stops the womb lining from being shed so that the pregnancy can continue developing.

Menstruation

If pregnancy does not occur, the corpus luteum does not receive its hCG signal. It therefore starts to degenerate around 10 days after ovulation and production of oestrogen and progesterone rapidly shuts down. Once the corpus luteum stops functioning, menstruation is triggered 3–4 days later, when arteries supplying the outer two-thirds of the endometrium go into spasm. This reduces their blood supply and starves the womb lining of oxygen so that it starts to break down. The womb starts to contract rhythmically and the outer two thirds of the endometrium are shed as a normal period – the inner third remains and will regenerate to produce a new womb lining during the next cycle. Menstruation usually starts approximately 14 days after ovulation. In the mean time, the remains of the corpus luteum cyst are eventually replaced by scar tissue.

By the end of a period, blood levels of the two ovarian hormones, oestrogen and progesterone, are at their lowest. This triggers production of GnRH, FSH and LH to start the next menstrual cycle.

MENSTRUAL FACTS

■ The average age at which periods start (menarche) is 13.4 years.
■ The average age when periods stop (the menopause) is 51 years.
■ From puberty until the menopause, women experience an average of 13 menstrual bleeds per year.
■ Allowing for the lack of periods during pregnancy, the average woman experiences between 400 and 500 periods during her lifetime.
■ The length of the menstrual cycle varies, with anything between 21 and 35 days considered normal.

- For some women, the interval between periods may be 15 days or less, and in others 50 days or more.
- The 28-day cycle usually quoted as the average only occurs in around 12 per cent of women.
- A period usually lasts from 1 to 8 days, with 3–5 days being most common.
- Ovulation usually occurs 13–15 days before the next period starts.
- The amount of menstrual fluid produced during a normal period varies between 30 ml and 75 ml. Therefore, throughout a woman's life, she experiences a total menstrual fluid loss of between 13.5 and 33.75 litres.

Regulation of Female Reproduction

Nearly all processes of female reproduction are regulated by progesterone and oestrogen acting together. This can only occur when the two hormones are made in the right quantities and at the right time in a woman's cycle. Like other hormones, oestrogen and progesterone travel round the body in the bloodstream until they recognize and interact with one of their special receptors on the wall of a body cell. The hormone then enters that cell and travels to the cell nucleus, where it switches on certain genes. This triggers production of one or more proteins, including enzymes, to produce effects linked with either oestrogen or progesterone.

Oestrogens

The ovaries produce several different female hormones which have a similar action and are together referred to as oestrogens. These include:

- oestradiol – the most potent form of oestrogen
- oestrone
- oestriol – the weakest oestrogen.

Oestrogens are made by the cells lining your ovarian follicles (theca interna and granulosa cells), by the corpus luteum and – in pregnancy – by the placenta.

After producing their actions in the body, these hormones

are broken down in the liver to form a variety of weaker oestrogens. Some of these are excreted into your bile and then reabsorbed from the gut into your bloodstream. From the blood, unwanted oestrogen hormones are filtered out into your urine (10 different breakdown products of oestrogen can be identified in your urine). Oestrogens stimulate many body tissues, including the:

- uterus
- breasts
- bones
- heart
- blood vessels
- brain
- vagina
- vulva
- bladder
- urethra
- mucous membranes
- skin
- hair.

As well as helping to regulate the menstrual cycle, oestrogen has a number of other effects in your body. It can:

- stimulate growth of ovarian follicles
- stimulate growth of breasts
- increase production of new bone
- keep your tissues elastic – especially skin and blood vessel walls
- lower cholesterol levels and discourage hardening and furring up of the arteries
- increase blood flow to the uterus and the growth of uterine muscle cells
- increase the motility of the Fallopian tubes
- maintain female body shape and patterns of fat storage
- help to regulate your sex drive
- keep mucous membranes moist

- thin down secretions of sebaceous glands, making blackheads and spots less likely.

Progesterone

The word *progesterone* comes from the Latin *pro* and *gestatio*, meaning *for pregnancy*. Progesterone is mainly secreted by the dominant follicle just before ovulation, and by the corpus luteum in the second half of the menstrual cycle. Blood levels of progesterone are highest during the third week of your menstrual cycle, then start to fall as the corpus luteum fails (if a fertilized egg implants it produces human Chorionic Gonadotrophin to keep the corpus luteum going, in which case progesterone levels increase).

Progesterone acts on three main body tissues:

1. uterus
2. breasts
3. brain.

Progesterone has several important effects in your body:

- changes the growth phase of the womb lining to the secretory phase in preparation for receiving a fertilized egg
- maintains early pregnancy by preventing menstruation
- acts together with oestrogen to support the production of breastmilk
- relaxes smooth muscle cells in the uterus and elsewhere
- prevents production of leutinizing hormone (LH) from the pituitary gland – this prevents ovulation during pregnancy and, to some extent, during breastfeeding
- changes cervical and vaginal mucus after ovulation, so that conception is less likely once a released egg has started to mature
- encourages salt and fluid retention (which is linked with pre-menstrual symptoms in some women).

ABNORMAL MENSTRUATION AROUND THE TIME

OF THE MENOPAUSE

As the menopause approaches, some women continue to have normal, regular periods, like clockwork, which then suddenly stop. It is more common, however, to notice gradual changes in your periods. Your menstrual pattern may become:

- irregular with no fixed pattern
- more frequent
- less frequent
- heavier than usual
- lighter than normal

You should tell your doctor straightaway if you notice:

- bleeding after intercourse
- unexpected bleeding (spotting) in between your periods
- post-menopausal bleeding.

Irregular Menstrual Bleeding

Periods may come more frequently than normal (for example, every 21 days or less) or less often (every two to three months). The most common cause of an irregular cycle around the menopause is that, as your ovaries run out of eggs, ovulation fails to occur in some cycles. When ovulation fails, there is no empty follicle to develop into the corpus luteum and secrete progesterone hormone. Ovarian oestrogens continue to stimulate growth of your womb lining (endometrium), however, so the proliferative phase of your menstrual cycle carries on without switching to the secretory phase. Soon the endometrium becomes so thick that it outgrows its blood supply. It then becomes starved of oxygen and starts to break down, triggering what seems like a normal, if early, menstrual bleed. The time taken for bleeding to occur is variable but is usually less than 28 days from the onset of the previous period. Bleeding also varies from scanty to profuse. Other possible causes of irregular – especially infrequent – periods are:

- stress
- pregnancy
- being very overweight or significantly underweight
- an overactive or underactive thyroid gland
- stopping the oral contraceptive Pill
- general illness
- polycystic ovaries (multiple small cysts on the ovaries)
- hormone imbalances.

Even if your periods aren't painful and aren't really troubling you, if they are irregular this may indicate an underlying condition – apart from approaching menopause – that needs treating. All cases are therefore worth bringing to your doctor's attention.

Heavy Periods

A heavy period can last for 10 days or longer, with flooding and sometimes clots.

One in 10 women suffers from heavy periods (menorrhagia) at some time during her life – especially around the time of the menopause. A common cause is lack of ovulation, so that the endometrium plumps up excessively leading to a heavy period as well as an irregular one. Other causes of heavy periods at this time of life include:

- fibroids (knot-like swellings in womb muscle)
- uterine polyps
- endometriosis (womb lining cells found outside the womb cavity)
- pelvic inflammatory disease (infection of the upper reproductive tract)
- rarely, cancer of the cervix, endometrium or ovary

If you suffer from heavy periods, you should take a supplement containing iron and consult your doctor in case investigation and treatment are needed. If heavy bleeding is allowed to continue, it can lead to anaemia and, in extreme cases, may even trigger angina (heart pain).

Painful Periods

The lining of the womb (endometrium) makes hormone-like chemicals called prostaglandins. These help the womb to contract during a period to control bleeding. Some women suffer from excessive pain (dysmenorrhoea) which usually starts with the onset of bleeding and lasts from several hours to several days. It tends to be spasmodic or colicky in nature and may be accompanied by diarrhoea, nausea and even vomiting. If pain is excessive, consult your doctor as you may need investigation for problems such as fibroids or endometriosis.

Pre-menstrual Syndrome

Pre-menstrual syndrome (PMS) is a common and distressing problem affecting as many as one in two women. It often becomes worse around the time of the menopause and may be prolonged when periods are missed or delayed. Usually, the symptoms of PMS start in the two weeks before a period is due and stop quickly once bleeding occurs. Even if your hormone levels are too low to trigger a period, they can still cause symptoms of PMS, such as:

- depression
- anxiety
- irritability
- poor concentration
- tiredness
- bingeing
- bloating
- breast tenderness
- headache and backache.

PMS is thought to be due to a relative imbalance between oestrogen and progesterone – something that usually becomes more pronounced as the menopause approaches.

Some research suggests that progesterone can't work properly when blood sugar levels are low. Nibbling regular carbohydrate snacks every 3 hours can help to reduce symptoms. Evening Primrose Oil contains hormone building-blocks and will help to even out hormonal imbalances, but needs to be taken at doses of up to 3 g a day for at least three months before an effect may be noticed. Also cut down on intakes of salt, alcohol, caffeine, eat a wholefood diet and try to keep as physically active as possible.

Menstrual Chart

If your periods are causing problems around the menopause, it is worth keeping a menstrual diary like the one below, which you can show to your doctor. This will help you keep track of when you bleed or have PMS-like symptoms. Start with the first month on the first day of your period (Day 1) and begin a new line for each period. Use different symbols for different events. In the table below, o = spotting, x = light bleeding, h = heavy bleeding, f = hot flushes, d = depression, i = irritability, p = pain, t = tiredness, b = bloating and s = symptom-free.

DAYS OF CYCLE

Month	1	2	3	4	5	6	7	8	9	10	11	12	13	14	15	16	17	18	19	20	21	22	23	24	25	26	27	28	29	30
1	x	x	h	h	h	h	h	x	s	s	s	s	s	s	s	d	i	d	i	f	b	d	b	b	o	o	–	–	–	–
2																														
3																														

Post-Menopausal Bleeding

Most women breathe a sigh of relief when the menopause approaches and their periods stop. Any vaginal bleeding appearing more than six months after you thought your periods had stopped should not be dismissed out of hand. Always tell your doctor if you notice post-menopausal bleeding (PMB). Bleeding occurring more than 12 months after your last period – even if it's only a little spotting – needs investigation as a matter of urgency. In nine out of 10 cases, nothing abnormal will be found, so try not to panic. One per cent of single episodes of PMB and 10 per cent of recurrent PMB may be due to cancer, however – if caught early your chances of successful treatment are much better.

PMB can occur when a doctor prescribes HRT but forgets to warn the woman that her monthly period may return. Other causes include:

- general thinning of tissues due to lack of oestrogen
- trauma during intercourse – especially after a time of sexual abstinence
- a polyp (benign fleshy growth) of the cervix or endometrium
- fibroids – benign tumours of uterine muscle
- over-stimulation of the endometrium (cystic hyperplasia) due to excessive doses of oestrogen (for example, where oestrogen HRT but no progestogen is taken by a woman who has not had a hysterectomy) – *see Chapter* 7
- cancer of the cervix, endometrium or ovaries
- rarely, a hormone-secreting tumour elsewhere in the body, which may stimulate the womb and cause PMB.

Although this list may seem frightening, it is important to have PMB checked out – in the majority of cases no cause is found, but if there is a serious reason early treatment often results in a cure.

Chapter Three

TRIGGERS AND SYMPTOMS OF THE MENOPAUSE

WHAT TRIGGERS THE MENOPAUSE?

The process leading up to the menopause begins when your ovaries start running out of eggs. While a woman has around half a million eggs at the time of puberty, these disappear or stop responding to hormone signals at an average rate of around 1,000–1,500 per month. On top of this, around 15 eggs start to develop and mature during each monthly cycle, but only one – from the dominant follicle – is usually released at ovulation (*see page* 7). At some stage during the age range 45–55, a woman's supply of eggs will have dwindled to the extent that an irregular number start developing each month.

Oestrogen hormone is mainly produced by cells lining the ovarian follicles. As the ovaries start to run out of eggs, and as the follicles that are left disintegrate or age and stop responding to hormone signals, oestrogen levels gradually fall. The pituitary gland senses this and tries to kick-start the tiring ovaries by increasing its secretion of follicle stimulating hormone (FSH) and leutinizing hormone (LH). Both of these are thought to contribute to menopausal symptoms such as hot flushes and night sweats.

As oestrogen levels fall, the womb lining (endometrium) loses its main source of stimulation. In many cases, while the ovaries produce enough oestrogen to stimulate growth of the womb lining, it is not enough to trigger ovulation. As a result, periods become irregular, and may be unusually heavy or unusually light. Your periods will eventually stop at the menopause proper, when the ovaries finally run out of eggs. The average age at which this happens is 51 years.

For some women, the menopause occurs before the age of 44. This is classed as a premature menopause (some doctors use 40 as the cut-off age); rarely, it may occur as early as the teens. There are cases where a young girl suffers from hot flushes and menopausal symptoms almost as soon as her periods first start, although this is rare.

For most women, the age at which her mother reached the menopause is a good guide to when she will go through it her-self. A few other factors also determine when your menopause will occur – for example whether you smoke, are under stress or have had a partial hysterectomy (even though your ovaries were left intact).

Smoking Cigarettes and the Menopause

The more you smoke, the sooner your periods cease – heavy smokers can reach the menopause two years earlier than non-smokers. Several chemicals found in cigarette smoke (such as nicotine, arabinase, conitine) interfere with enzymes that process oestrogen hormone. Smoking both reduces the amount of oestrogen produced, and increases the rate at which it is broken down. This lowers blood oestrogen levels enough to trigger an earlier menopause than usual.

Stress and the Menopause

Psychological factors can affect the menstrual cycle, and it is well known that when a woman is under stress she may miss a period. Similarly, it seems that stress can in some cases trigger the menopause, although this is poorly understood. Traumatic events such as illness, severe financial problems, or the death of a close relative can all be followed by a sudden stopping of periods.

Premature Menopause

If your menopause occurs before the age of 44, it is classified as premature. A natural premature menopause affects around 1 in 100 women. It is often triggered when the immune system for some reason starts to make antibodies against the ovaries – in effect, the body is attacking part of itself which it has misinterpreted as foreign tissue. In other women there is a genetic link: it may be that they have inherited fewer egg follicles, or follicles which have a shorter than normal life span.

It has been estimated that 8 per cent of women experience a premature menopause under the age of 40 as a result of medical or surgical treatment. When added to those naturally experiencing a premature menopause, as many as 1 in 12 women enters the menopause before the age of 40.

There is some evidence that a woman who has an early menopause is more at risk of developing coronary heart disease (CHD), stroke and dementia in the future, as oestrogen helps to keep blood vessels elastic and protects against these diseases (*see page 84*).

Hysterectomy and the Menopause

It is estimated that one in five women will have a hysterectomy or removal of her womb lining (endometrial resection or ablation) by the age of 55. The usual reason is that periods have become unacceptably heavy, prolonged or painful.

Different surgeons have different approaches to removing or conserving the ovaries during hysterectomy. The disadvantage of having the ovaries out is that you will have an instant, surgically-induced menopause, which usually produces severe symptoms unless HRT is started quickly. The advantage of having your ovaries removed – especially as the menopause approaches – is that you will never develop ovarian cancer. This is an important point, as it is estimated that 1 in 500 women whose ovaries are left inside will eventually develop an ovarian malignancy. Even where your ovaries are left intact:

- 1 in 4 women develop menopausal symptoms within two years
- on average, you will go through the menopause 4 years earlier – around the age of 47 – than a woman who has not had a hysterectomy

The most likely reason is that the operation reduces ovarian blood supply. Alternatively, there may be some as yet unrecognized interaction between the ovaries and uterus which causes the ovaries to fail more quickly once a hysterectomy is performed.

REASONS WHY HYSTERECTOMY MAY BE PERFORMED

- excessive menstrual bleeding (menorrhagia)
- fibroids (benign tumours of muscle in the womb wall)
- endometriosis (where womb lining cells are found outside their usual site, causing pain or bleeding)
- pelvic inflammatory disease (infection and inflammation of the upper female reproductive tract)
- prolapse of the womb
- pelvic cancer (for example of the cervix, endometrium or ovaries).

Drug-induced Menopause

Some types of medical drug treatment may temporarily or permanently affect the ovaries to produce menopausal symptoms. These include false menopause drugs (such as danazol, GnRH inhibitors) anti-oestrogen drugs (tamoxifen, for example) and chemotherapy agents.

Danazol

Treatment with danazol triggers a reversible, temporary menopause. It is a synthetic form of the male hormone, testosterone, and is used to treat a number of gynaecological conditions, including endometriosis, fibrocystic breast disease, heavy periods (menorrhagia) and pre-menstrual syndrome.

Danazol works directly on the ovaries to interfere with the enzymes responsible for the production of oestrogen and progesterone, and also affects the hypothalamus to lower the secretion of gonadotrophin releasing hormone (GnRH – *see page 5*). This results in lowered oestrogen levels – similar to those found after the menopause. Danazol is therefore classed as a reversible, pseudomenopausal (false menopause) drug. While taking it, the ovaries stop making oestrogen and eggs stop ripening.

Three out of four women taking danazol will notice several body changes, of which many mimic the symptoms of the menopause, while others are due to changing from a female hormone environment to a more masculine one. Common effects include:

- stopping of periods (amenorrhoea)
- hot flushes and sweating
- mood changes
- shrinking breasts
- tiredness
- lowered sex drive
- depression
- weight gain
- muscle development
- oily skin
- fluid retention
- acne
- hairiness.

Once danazol is stopped, periods usually return to normal within 3 to 8 weeks and the false menopause symptoms disappear.

GnRH Analogues

A group of drugs called the GnRH analogues also produce a reversible, false menopause, and are used to treat a few gynaecological conditions such as endometriosis and breast cancer. The drugs work by interfering with production of gonadotrophin releasing hormone (GnRH) in the hypothalamus. GnRH is what triggers secretion of FSH and LH from the pituitary gland; these two hormones in turn act on the ovary to stimulate production of oestrogen and progesterone (*see Chapter 2*).

GnRH analogues bind to the pituitary gland at the sites (receptors) where GnRH usually triggers its action. But instead of quickly dropping off to free up the receptor again, as natural GnRH does, the drug sits on its receptors for 3–8 hours. When the drug first binds to the receptors, it stimulates production of FSH and LH, but as it continues to sit there, the pituitary gland becomes over-stimulated and drained so that it stops making both FSH and LH. Levels of FSH and LH start to go up for 3 to 10 days before starting to go down, and a reversible, false menopause is usually triggered after about 2 weeks.

GnRH analogues cannot be given by mouth as they are quickly broken down by digestive juices before they have an effect. They are therefore given in the form of a nasal spray, or injection under the skin (subcutaneous). Four GnRH analogues are currently in use to treat endometriosis:

1. buserelin
2. goserelin
3. leuprorelin
4. nafarelin.

Two other drugs, tryptorelin and histrelin, are also under investigation and may become available in the future.

Because they produce a false menopause, GnRH analogues can trigger menopausal symptoms that include:

■ hot flushes
■ sweats
■ lowered sex drive
■ acne
■ oily hair/skin
■ vaginal dryness
■ reduced breast size
■ mood swings.

They are so effective in producing an artificial menopause that they can also produce long-term effects of thinning bones (osteoporosis) and increased risk of heart attack. Treatment with GnRH analogues is therefore usually restricted to a single 6-month course, except in special circumstances.

One possible solution is to add back some oestrogen or progesterone to prevent this happening, or to combine a small dose of danazol with the GnRH agonists, as danazol helps to increase bone density slightly.

Most women usually restart their periods within 6 to 8 weeks of stopping treatment. Rarely, a woman using a GnRH analogue may enter the menopause while on treatment and not restart her periods once therapy stops.

Anti-oestrogen Drugs

A group of drugs that block the action of oestrogen hormone are used to treat some hormone-responsive gynaecological conditions such as breast cancer. When given to pre-menopausal women, they sometimes produce a reversible loss of periods (amenorrhoea) and menopause-like symptoms such as hot flushes. Tamoxifen is one such drug.

Chemotherapy Drugs

Chemotherapy and/or radiotherapy to treat cancer can temporarily or permanently affect the ovaries and may trigger an early menopause. Younger women have a better chance of their ovaries recovering than older women, but this will usually depend on the type of treatment given; any risk will be discussed fully with the woman before she decides whether or not to go ahead. It is usually possible for a section of ovarian tissue, complete with egg follicles, to be removed and frozen before treatment. This gives the woman a chance of having fertility treatment using her own eggs in the future.

Tests and Investigations to Confirm the Menopause

A blood test to measure levels of FSH and LH from the pituitary gland can show whether you are approaching the menopause or not.

These hormones are produced by the pituitary gland to stimulate egg and hormone production in the ovaries. Levels of FSH and LH usually peak in the middle of your cycle, just before ovulation occurs. As your ovaries produce less and less oestrogen as the menopause approaches, your pituitary gland increases its output of FSH and LH in an attempt to boost ovarian action. When FSH and LH reach a certain level, they are said to be in the 'menopausal range' as the ovary is obviously no longer responding to the usual signals. The following blood levels taken together are usually diagnostic of the menopause:

- an FSH level above 25 U/l
- an LH level above 50 U/l and
- an oestradiol (oestrogen) level of less than 150 pmol/l.

Occasionally, some women with FSH and LH levels in the menopausal range will return to a normal menstrual cycle if the ovaries suddenly start responding to FSH and LH again. This is not common, but a woman cannot assume that she is no longer fertile. As pregnancy can sometimes occur during the year or two after the last menstrual period, so you still need to use an effective method of contraception (*see page 57*).

PHYSICAL SYMPTOMS OF THE MENOPAUSE

In the 5–10 years leading up to the actual menopause (the date of your last period), your body starts going through a variety of changes. As oestrogen levels fall, tissues that are responsive to the hormone lose an important source of stimulation. These tissues include your:

- vagina
- vulva
- uterus
- breasts
- bones
- heart
- blood vessels
- brain
- urethra
- bladder
- skin
- mucous membranes
- hair.

The rate at which oestrogen levels fall helps to determine how bad your symptoms are. If your oestrogen levels fall off relatively slowly, your body is designed to cope with what is a normal biological event, so that you do not suffer unduly. If your hormone levels fall quickly, however, your body has little time to adapt and you are plunged into the deep end of the changes occurring as a result of oestrogen withdrawal.

The Adrenal Glands

Usually, up to 5 per cent of circulating sex hormones are made by your adrenal glands. As your ovaries stop working, your adrenal glands take over some of their function and produce small amounts of oestrogen as well as doubling their output of testosterone-like male hormones (androgens). Some of these androgens have a weak oestrogen-like action. They can also be converted into oestrogen by other tissues in your body, especially your stores of fat. As a result, heavier women who have more fat stores seem less likely to suffer from severe menopausal symptoms than women who are slim.

If you have been under long-term stress, however, your adrenal glands may already be working full blast producing stress hormones such as adrenaline. When your menopause approaches, they have no extra reserves to boost their output of sex hormones. Stressed women tend to suffer more and worse menopausal symptoms than women whose lives are less stressful. They are also more likely to lose their sex drive. *For advice on coping with stress, see Chapter 6.*

Not every woman experiences problems around the menopause:

■ 25 per cent of women have few if any symptoms
■ 50 per cent of women experience only mild symptoms
■ 25 per cent of women, however, suffer dreadfully.

In 4 out of 5 women who experience symptoms, these last for more than 1 year. For some women, symptoms last more than 5 years.

The physical symptoms of the menopause fall into two main groups: those due to the sudden withdrawal of oestrogen hormone, and those which occur partly as a result of getting older, which are less directly linked to hormone levels.

Menopausal Symptoms due to Oestrogen Withdrawal

Symptoms that are directly due to falling oestrogen levels include:

- hot flushes
- night sweats
- difficulty sleeping
- vaginal dryness and difficulties with intercourse, including loss of sex drive
- bladder problems
- loss of skin sensitivity
- migraine.

Hot Flushes

Hot flushes are the most common menopausal symptom, experienced by around 80 per cent of women.

Women who suffer from hot flushes seem to be more sensitive to lowered oestrogen levels than women who do not flush, and tend to develop more menopausal symptoms overall than those who do not flush. They may come on early in the peri-menopausal period, before you have noticed any changes in your periods. In some women, they only occur over a short time, coinciding with a larger than usual fluctuation in hormone levels. In most cases, the tendency towards hot flushes passes within 1 or 2 years, although it may last for 5 years or more.

Each hot flush usually lasts from 1–5 minutes, although occasionally one may last an hour or more. Some women suffer at least 1 per day, while others may only get 1 per week. A few unlucky women seem to get several per hour – some claim to suffer as many as 50 hot flushes in a day, though it is unusual to have them this badly. Few women suffer more than 12 hot flushes per day.

The flush is usually felt over the upper trunk, neck, face and arms. Blood vessels in the skin dilate to increase blood flow so that your skin becomes red and hot. Skin temperature rises by

1–4°C – enough to make you feel sweaty and uncomfortable, although your internal body temperature stays much the same.

By opening up blood vessels in your skin, your heart has to work harder to pump blood around your circulation, so your pulse rate usually goes up. Many women also have a premonition that the flush is on its way, and may feel unusually anxious, unwell, or notice sensations of skin tingling, prickling, pins and needles or pressure in their head. Others may feel dizzy and light-headed as their blood vessels dilate and blood pressure goes down.

Hot flushes can be triggered by a number of factors, including:

- hot surroundings – wearing heavy clothes, central heating, summer
- increased humidity
- alcohol
- caffeine
- eating hot food or drinking hot drinks
- eating spicy foods
- exposure to cigarette smoke
- strong emotions
- stress
- tiredness
- some drugs.

One of the worst things about a hot flush is that it is such a visible sign that you are suffering a menopausal problem. Unfortunately, worrying about having a flush in public is likely to bring one on and/or make it worse.

Researchers are still unsure of the exact cause of a hot flush. It was thought to be linked with increased levels of FSH and LH, as just before a flush there seems to be a surge of activity in the hypothalamus which releases GnRH – but no definite link between hormone levels and hot flushes has been found.

The most popular current theory is that hot flushes are due to changes in the metabolism of a brain chemical (noradrenaline) produced by falling levels of oestrogen. This affects the setting of the body's thermostat, which is regulated in the hypothalamus in the brain – next door to where GnRH is produced. Noradrenaline is also affected by stress, which is probably why stress can trigger a hot flush.

The body's responses to excessive heat or cold are regulated by different parts of the hypothalamus:

1. Stimulation of the front (anterior) part of the hypothalamus causes flushing and sweating and, in extreme cases, can reset the body's thermostat from 37°C to as much as 43°C (as during a fever).
2. Stimulation of the back (posterior) part of the hypothalamus produces shivering.

Special cells making GnRH are sandwiched between these two areas. For some reason, the temperature regulation system does not work very well when oestrogen levels are lower than normal. It may be that, as cells in the hypothalamus make more and more GnRH to trigger release of FSH and LH from the pituitary gland (in an attempt to kick-start the failing ovaries), the nearby temperature regulation system is over-stimulated.

If you develop a flush, don't be embarrassed. Breathe in deeply, sit still and try to relax. It can help to stand near an open window, drink a chilled drink, use a personal battery-operated fan or suck an ice-cube or ice cream. A small packet of wet wipes in your handbag will help to cool you down until you can wash or shower to freshen up.

Night Sweats

Hot flushes are often followed by profuse sweating, especially at night. Typically, you may wake up sweating, with a feeling that you can't breathe. You may be so drenched in sweat that you need to change your night-clothes and bed linen. Some women suffer from cold sweats rather than hot sweats and feel clammy and chilled. More usually, feelings of hot and cold alternate. As the body heats up, sweating occurs to cool you down again and is often so successful that you soon start shivering and pulling the covers back over yourself.

Researchers are unsure why bad hot flushes and sweats seem to occur at night. The activity of your hypothalamus and pituitary gland seems to peak at night between 1 and 3 a.m., but there is no proven link between your hormone levels and the occurrence of night sweats.

If you are awoken at night with a sweat or flush, you may be one of the lucky ones who is able to freshen up then go straight back to sleep. More usually, you will lie there tossing and turning and find sleep difficult, or will sleep only briefly before waking up again.

If you fall into the sleep difficulty pattern, you are likely to become deficient in REM (rapid eye movement) sleep and end up feeling exhausted during the day. This can also lead to depression. Hormone replacement therapy (HRT) has been shown to increase the time a woman spends in REM sleep. See page 157 for self-help tips on how to sleep better.

One of the most useful aids for a night sweat is to have a 20- to 30 cm office fan by the side of your bed – flinging off the bed clothes and switching on a cool breeze will soon make you feel more comfortable. Keeping a bottle of chilled mineral water in the bedroom (in a wine cooler, for instance) will also help you to freshen up.

YOUR TEMPERATURE REGULATION MECHANISMS

EFFECTS OF HEAT

- flushing – dilation of veins in the skin so heat radiates off you
- sweating – heat is used up as sweat evaporates
- increased breathing rate – so you literally blow heat off
- loss of appetite – to slow production of heat during digestion
- sluggish behaviour – to slow production of heat during physical activity.

EFFECTS OF COLD

- shivering – to generate heat through muscle action
- hunger – to produce heat during digestion
- increased activity levels – to make heat through physical exertion such as stamping feet
- increased production of noradrenaline and adrenaline – to stimulate temperature regulation in the hypothalamus and boost your metabolic rate
- shutting down of blood vessels in the skin – to conserve heat
- curling up – to reduce body surface and conserve heat radiation
- goosebumps – hair on skin stands on end to trap body warmth.

Difficulty Sleeping

Even if you don't have sleep problems due to hot flushes or night sweats, you may develop insomnia due to oestrogen withdrawal.

Sleep is a form of unconsciousness which is your natural state of rest. This is essential for physical and mental well-being, as it is a time of rest, rejuvenation and regeneration. Growth hormone is secreted in increased amounts during sleep, muscles and joints recover from constant use during the day, and most of the body's repair work is carried out – more skin, red blood cells, immune cells, intestinal lining cells and hair follicle cells are produced during sleep than when you are awake. Protein in all parts of the body is replenished faster during sleep as well, yet there is no conclusive evidence that sleep is essential for any body organ except the brain. Even here, researchers are stumped as, paradoxically, the brain is actually more active during sleep than when you are wide awake.

The brain contains oestrogen receptors, and the menopause does affect your natural sleep pattern. There are two main types of sleep:

1. Rapid Eye Movement (REM) sleep, in which the eyes are constantly on the move.
2. Slow Wave (or non-REM sleep), in which the eyes are relatively still.

There are four stages of slow wave sleep – the lightest is stage 1 and the deepest, stage 4. When you first fall asleep, you rapidly pass through stages 1 and 2, then spend 70–100 minutes in stages 3 and 4. Sleep then lightens and a short period of around 10 minutes' REM follows. This cycle repeats 4 to 6 times throughout the night, but as morning approaches more and more time – up to 1 hour – is spent in REM sleep.

Interestingly, people who only sleep 5 hours per night tend to get a similar amount of slow wave sleep as those who regularly sleep 8 hours per night – additional time spent sleeping is spent in REM sleep.

On average, you spend the following amount of time in each stage of sleep:

Stage 1	5 per cent of the night (light sleep)
Stage 2	50 per cent of the night
Stage 3	5 per cent of the night
Stage 4	15 per cent of the night (deep sleep)
REM	25 per cent.

Your sleep pattern naturally changes throughout life. As you get older, you spend less and less time in stage 4 (really deep) sleep, so that by the age of 70 most people get no stage 4 sleep at all. As sleep tends to be light, it is common for the elderly to wake several times during the night, though they may not recall this next morning. Researchers have recently found that low oestrogen levels are linked with having less REM sleep, although the women affected are not necessarily sleep deprived. Sleep problems are usually helped by HRT, which also improves your sleep structure, increasing the amount of time you spend in REM sleep.

Other common sleep problems around the time of the menopause include waking too early or having difficulty going off to sleep in the first place. Early morning waking is one of the biological symptoms of depression, so if you also feel low in mood and burst into tears easily, it is important to seek help (*see* Psychological Symptoms of the Menopause, *page 41*).

Vaginal Dryness
Vaginal dryness is usually a relatively late symptom which can come on a year or more after you first developed other problems.

Over half of all women develop vaginal dryness and lack of lubrication after the menopause that is bad enough to need treatment. This is because oestrogen is needed to switch on secretion of vaginal lubrication. Sex may become uncomfortable or painful and may even result in bleeding from thinning tissues. Most women notice some difficulties with intercourse, including loss of sex drive (*see Chapter 4*).

Eventually, vaginal tissues – including the clitoris – will shrink (atrophy), which can have a devastating effect on your sex life. Using local oestrogen creams/gels or taking HRT will reverse and overcome these changes.

Bladder Problems

The tissues of the bladder and urethra (tube through which urine flows from the bladder to the outside) are also sensitive to oestrogen. As a result, many menopausal women develop symptoms such as:

- wanting to run to the loo more often than usual (frequency)
- having to rush to the loo to pass urine (urgency)
- passing only small amounts of urine
- leaking of urine (stress incontinence – *see Chapter 5*)
- increased risk of bladder infection (cystitis).

Most of these problems can be overcome with pelvic floor exercises, HRT or diet and lifestyle changes.

As the bladder symptoms of oestrogen withdrawal are similar to those of infection (cystitis), it can be difficult to know which is causing your problem. In general, if passing urine stings or burns, if your urine smells unpleasant, or if you notice blood in your urine, an infective cystitis is likely. If in doubt, always seek medical advice, and take a sample of urine along to the surgery with you. This can be tested with reagent dipsticks to look for signs of bacterial infection.

Loss of Skin Sensitivity

Your skin loses some of its sensitivity when oestrogen levels fall. This can also interfere with your enjoyment of sex – *see page 50*.

Migraine

As oestrogen has such a profound effect on blood vessels through-out your body – especially small ones – migraine is three times more common in women than men. Lots of women find they develop migraine for the first time during the menopause, which then improves as oestrogen-withdrawal symptoms fade away.

Migraine affects 1 in 10 people generally. Attacks usually begin around puberty, then strike intermittently until middle age. Three quarters of all sufferers are aged between 16 and 45. For some sufferers, however, symptoms continue into old age. The average non-menopausal sufferer experiences 13 attacks per year, each lasting around 18 hours. During the menopause, however, you may only have a few attacks.

There are several different sorts of migraine:

- *migraine without aura* – or common migraine – consists of a severe, throbbing, pulsating or hammering headache on one side, usually with abdominal symptoms. These include loss of appetite, nausea, vomiting, dislike of food, constipation or diarrhoea. Nine out of 10 sufferers experience this form of migraine.
- *migraine with aura* – or classic migraine – includes visual disturbances as well as any or all of the symptoms of common migraine. Vision can be distorted, with shimmering or flashing lights, strange zig-zag shapes or blind spots. One in 10 sufferers gets this form of migraine.
- In some rare forms of migraine, pins and needles, numbness or temporary paralysis may occur down one side of the body.

The exact cause of migraine is not fully understood. Attacks seem to be linked to chemical changes in the blood vessel walls and nerve cells within the skull. The most important chemical involved is called serotonin (5-hydroxytryptamine, or 5HT for short). Migraine headache occurs when blood vessels widen so that tissues become congested. Serotonin is in short supply during this phase. Some sufferers find their migraine is triggered by certain factors, such as:

- stress or relief of stress (as at the end of a long, trying week)
- physical fatigue or lack of sleep (due, for example, to hot sweats, insomnia)
- certain foods – such as cheese, alcohol – especially red wine, chocolate
- extreme emotions – such as menopausal mood swings
- hormonal changes, for example those caused by menstruation, the oral contraceptive Pill, menopausal symptoms.

Migraine is usually only felt on one side of the head or is worse on one side (unilateral). It often centres around one eye and is accompanied by abdominal and/or visual symptoms. In contrast, a tension headache is a severe, continuous pressure felt on both sides of the head (bilateral). It can be felt over the top of the skull (vertex), over the back of the head (occiput) or above both eyes. It may feel like a tight, constricting band, or a non-specific ache. Tension head-aches can occur at any age, but are also more common around the time of the menopause. They are linked with stress and depression.

Migraine without aura is often misdiagnosed as a tension headache. If you think your recurrent headache may be migraine, it is important to tell your doctor.

Several different migraine treatments are now available – some over the counter, others by prescription only. While some people find simple analgesics control their symptoms, others need stronger medication. It's worth noting that digestion often shuts down during a migraine attack, so tablets are not always well absorbed. You may find that soluble or effervescent formulations suit you best.

There are two approaches to migraine treatment: the short-term relief of an acute attack, and long-term preventative (prophylactic) treatment for people with frequent, disabling symptoms.

Short-term treatments contain simple painkillers such as aspirin, paracetamol or codeine. Some also contain an antiemetic to stop you feeling sick. The most modern treatments involve drugs that act on blood vessels in the brain in a similar way to serotonin to switch a migraine off in its early stages.

Long-term anti-migraine treatments come in several forms; if migraine has come on during the menopause, HRT may well be your best option in controlling attacks.

Other Symptoms that May Develop after the Menopause

Several physical changes occur in your body around the time of the menopause, partly as a normal result of getting older, although they are made worse by lack of oestrogen. Things you may notice include:

- wrinkling and thinning of skin/skin mottling and discoloration
- acne
- changes in hair texture and increased hair thinning
- increase in facial hair
- spreading waistline
- tiredness and lack of energy
- non-specific aches and pains.

Wrinkles and Skin Mottling

Every time your skin is exposed to the sun, it is damaged by ultraviolet rays. Over the years, this photodamage adds up to cause premature wrinkles and skin blemishes – a process known as photo-ageing or heliodermatitis. This is a normal part of the ageing process although you can avoid some of the effects by minimizing the exposure of your skin to the sun. Solar ultra-violet radiation consists of UVA and UVB rays. UVB causes sunburn and long-term changes responsible for skin ageing and skin cancer. UVA does not burn, but is responsible for photosensitivity reactions and also contributes to long-term photo-ageing.

As a result of photo-ageing, your skin cells are unable to regenerate normally and collagen fibres that provide underlying skin support become matted, branched and twisted. Skin that is exposed to the sun over a long period of time eventually becomes inelastic, thickened, yellow, scaly, blemished and wrinkled.

Your skin tissues are also sensitive to oestrogen, and after the menopause your skin will become thinner, drier and more fragile. You will develop skin mottling and discoloration at a faster rate, and may develop broken capillaries (telangiectasia) which look like fine wine-red spidery tracings, especially on your face.

Women who smoke cigarettes are five times more likely to suffer premature wrinkles than non-smokers, with the number of facial wrinkles directly linked to the number of cigarettes smoked.

There are three main types of skin wrinkle:

1. Crinkles – fine lines that disappear when skin is stretched. These are due to the breakdown of elastic fibres in your skin and start before the menopause, around the age of 30.
2. Glyphic wrinkles – accentuation of normal skin markings. Skin becomes yellowed and thickened where exposed to light – especially around the neck and eyes. These wrinkles become more pronounced after the menopause.
3. Linear furrows – grooves related to long-standing patterns of facial expression, whose positions are determined in childhood.

As well as wrinkles, ageing skin starts to develop other changes, including:

- age spots – areas of pigmentation on skin that has been exposed to light over many years. These are often seen on the backs of the hands, face and neck
- mottling – irregular pigmentation in which, paradoxically, the number of skin pigment cells (melanocytes) is actually decreased
- stellate pseudoscars – small spots that are white, star-shaped, and tend to appear after the age of 60
- guttate hypomelanoses – small round or angular spots that are pure white in colour and range in size from pinpoint to 15 mm across.
- ephelides – small, brown marks which darken in the sun
- senile lentigines – darkened patches of skin which can be over 1 cm across. They are often dark brown, but can also be yellow, light brown or even black

- pre-malignant lesions which can progress to skin cancer if not treated. There are three types of skin cancer: malignant melanoma, basal cell carcinoma, and squamous cell carcinoma. Malignant melanoma is now the second most common cancer in women (after cervical cancer).

If you notice any skin lesions that are enlarging, itching, scabbing, bleeding, changing in colour or in any other way, always seek medical advice. Caught early, most skin cancers are readily curable.

Acne

Although acne is usually thought of as a teenage problem, it can affect anyone of any age; studies suggest that 5 per cent of people in their forties suffer from acne-like spots. In some cases, skin outbreaks can come on after the menopause due to hormonal changes when levels of testosterone increase while levels of oestrogen fall.

Acne is thought to be triggered in some people by oversensitivity of skin oil (sebaceous) glands to normal blood levels of the male hormone, testosterone. Although this hypersensitivity usually starts in the teens and switches off again within a few years, some people have trouble-free skin until their late twenties, early thirties or at the menopause, and then suddenly develop spots.

When oil glands are overactive, they produce a thick, oily secretion known as sebum. If you have a type of bacteria called *Propionibacterium acnes* living on your skin, it can produce enzymes that break the sebum down into a variety of fatty acids. These, plus other effects of the bacteria on immune chemicals in your skin, trigger inflammation and lead to classic acne lesions in those who are sensitive to them.

If your skin starts to flare up after the menopause, don't be afraid to consult your GP for treatment. Unfortunately, acne treatment needs patience; often no benefits are seen for 6 to 8 weeks after starting therapy. It is important to keep up with the treatment, however, as after 2 months of continued and regular use, improvements of around 20 per cent per month are common. Treatment is usually needed for at least 6 months.

Hair Changes

The normal ageing process together with lack of oestrogen may make your hair feel drier and coarser than normal. You may also find that your hair is turning grey at a faster rate. Some women find that their skin and hair condition improve if they pay attention to their diet, take a good multinutrient supplement and increase their intake of essential fatty acids (found in Evening Primrose Oil and fish oils).

Increase in Facial Hair

Excess, unwanted hair is common. A quarter of all women have noticeable hair on their face, 15 per cent have hair on their chest, 30 per cent have it on their lower abdomen and 40 per cent on their thighs.

As levels of oestrogen fall around the time of the menopause, the effects of testosterone hormone become more pronounced, without the feminizing effects of oestrogen to counter-balance them. As a result, facial hair increases. By the age of 65, 40 per cent of women have a noticeable moustache and 10 per cent sprout hair on their chins. This is not due to any medically significant hormonal imbalance but to the changing balance between masculine and feminine hormones.

The best way to cope with unwanted hair is by using depilatory creams, plucking, epilation, waxing or – a more permanent method – having a course of electrolysis or laser treatment.

Electrolysis only works on growing hair, not on follicles in their rest phase, however, so you may find you need another course a few months later as resting follicles start to activate.

Contrary to popular belief, shaving does not thicken hair or make it grow faster. It does, however, slice off the tapered tip of the hair shaft to leave a flattened stubble that quickly becomes noticeable again.

Spreading Waistline

As you age, your metabolic rate naturally slows, sometimes by as much as 3 per cent per year. Between the ages of 27 and 47, your metabolic rate may fall by 12 per cent – this means you need to cut back on the number of calories you eat and increase your level of physical activity to avoid putting on weight. In practice, this often doesn't happen and the waist-line begins to spread. Between the ages of 25 and 70, the average woman:

- increases her body fat percentage from 27 per cent to 40 per cent
- loses 5 kg of lean body mass (muscle), which falls from an average of 40 kg to 35 kg

Falling levels of female sex hormones also mean you start to store excess fat differently than when you were younger. Rather than gaining weight on your breasts, hips and thighs, for example, you may develop a more male pattern of weight gain, putting on weight around your abdomen.

Overweight people who carry excess weight around their middle (apple-shaped) rather than around their hips (pear-shaped) are more at risk of hardening and furring up of the arteries, CHD, stroke, high blood pressure, high cholesterol levels and diabetes. This is probably due to the way your body handles dietary fats. If you are overweight and also apple-shaped, you have a higher risk of developing CHD – especially if this runs in your family. If you fall into this pattern of weight gain after the menopause, it is important to follow a low-fat diet and increase the amount of exercise you take (*see Chapter 9*).

Tiredness

Tiredness and lack of energy affect as many as 1 in 3 women during the menopausal years. It tends to creep up on you, making you feel washed out and exhausted for much of the time. These symptoms seem to be linked with oestrogen withdrawal as they usually improve with HRT, especially in women suffering more severe hot flushes. Minor deficiencies of vitamins and minerals may be involved, and women taking a good multinutrient supplement – including sensible levels of B group vitamins – usually notice an improvement.

Aches and Pains

Aches and pains are common during the time of oestrogen withdrawal. Headaches become more frequent and your joints and muscles may stiffen and hurt. It is possible that these symptoms are related to changes in blood flow and circulation in musculoskeletal tissues. Symptoms often improve with HRT.

PSYCHOLOGICAL SYMPTOMS

While many women expect to become emotional wrecks around the time of the menopause, this is far from usual – most cope well, with little in the way of emotional upheavals or depression. Having said that, when psychological symptoms do occur, they can be as devastating as the physical ones. Those that are most common include:

- irritability
- mood swings
- anxiety
- tearfulness and depression
- difficulty concentrating and poor memory.

Irritability

Irritability seems to be linked with falling oestrogen levels, which affect higher centres of the brain. This seems to be most common in women who have experienced irritability as a symptom of premenstrual syndrome, although some women who have never had problems before develop cyclical mood swings similar to PMS. In some cases, irritability is linked with lack of sleep, especially rapid eye movement (REM) sleep. Researchers have recently found that low oestrogen levels are linked with having less REM sleep, although the women affected are not necessarily sleep deprived. Lack of sleep can also be due to night sweats and hot flushes waking you up, or to general insomnia. Irritability usually gets better on its own, although HRT or complementary therapies (*see Chapter 8*) can help enormously.

Irritability can also be due to low blood sugar levels. It is worth drinking a glass of freshly squeezed orange juice for an instant lift, followed by a crispbread, slice of wholemeal bread, rice cake or banana to see if this helps (*see* Food Cravings, *page 40*).

Mood Swings

Some women going through the menopause experience alarming mood swings, going from happy to sad, or suffering from anxiety and panic attacks for no obvious reason. In contrast, other women find that once their periods stop they no longer suffer from pre-menstrual syndrome and actually feel more emotionally stable than before. While it is easy to blame emotional changes on falling hormone levels, this time of life is also one where you may be experiencing other stresses such as caring for elderly relatives, offspring leaving home, a husband in a mid-life crisis and your own changing self-image.

If your mood swings are pronounced, you may find it helps to take a regular energetic form of exercise such as going for a brisk walk or even taking up gentle jogging to get fit. Exercise releases chemicals in the brain that help to lift your mood and keep you on a more even keel. The exercise needs to be brisk enough to leave you slightly breathless and to raise your pulse to between 100–120 beats per minute.

If you are able to take HRT, this usually improves mood swings significantly – you will know if it is helping within 1–2 months.

Anxiety

Anxiety affects 5 per cent of the population and is associated with feelings of apprehension, dread and impending doom. It can cause physical symptoms similar to those caused by stress, such as:

- restlessness
- palpitations
- tremor
- flushing
- dizziness

- over-breathing (hyperventilation)
- loose bowels
- sweating – which makes hot flushes worse
- muscle tension
- difficulty sleeping.

In most cases, anxiety linked with other menopausal symptoms is self-limiting and gets better over the course of a few weeks without any specific treatment. Symptoms are usually made worse by drinking caffeine or alcohol, however, so it is worth avoiding these.

It is now thought that anxiety and panic attacks are linked with over-breathing (hyperventilation). As a result, you inhale too much oxygen and exhale too much carbon dioxide, causing an imbalance of respiratory gases which in turn makes your blood too alkaline. As well as triggering symptoms of dizziness, faintness and 'pins and needles' in the face and limbs, over-breathing sends messages to the brain that you are under stress and keeps the body on 'red alert'. Habitual hyperventilators may also experience chest pains, palpitations, sleep disturbances and other physical symptoms as well as anxiety. If you feel anxiety coming on, consciously try to slow and control your breathing – if necessary, the old trick of breathing in and out of a brown paper bag will do the trick – this helps you to breathe back in some of the carbon dioxide you have exhaled.

Tearfulness and Depression

Few people are blessed with a happy mood all the time. Most women are used to their mood going up and down almost with the weather. One day you may feel cheerful, energetic and lively, while the next you feel gloomy, listless and withdrawn for no obvious reason. These mood swings are a normal part of everyday life. But sometimes they can get out of hand – and if your mood swings too low, mild depression can occur.

Tearfulness is common around the time of the menopause, and is again linked with falling oestrogen levels. While mild cases usually improve rapidly with close support from family and friends, regular exercise and beneficial alternative treatments, in some cases your mood can fall even lower until you are suffering from a full-blown depressive illness.

Depression occurs when the level of various chemical messengers in the brain become unbalanced. These chemicals – known as neurotransmitters – are responsible for passing messages from one brain cell to another by passing across the tiny gap (synapse) between each brain cell. Once across the gap, they trigger an electrical response in the next brain cell to increase its activity. After it has done its job, the neurotransmitter is then reabsorbed into the cell that released it and broken down for re-cycling. If your neurotransmitter levels fall too low, messages are not passed from one brain cell to another properly and mild depression occurs – because your brain cells are not being kick-started like they should be.

Overall, women are twice as likely to suffer depression than men – your lifetime risk of developing a severe depressive illness is between 20 and 26 per cent, while for men it is 8 to 12 per cent. While it is traditionally believed that female depression is most likely to occur between the ages of 35 and 55 years – that is, in women approaching and just past the menopause – recent research suggests that female depression is no more common in your forties or fifties than earlier or later in life. For women who do develop depression around the time of the menopause, however, hormonal changes are the most usual trigger – to the extent that a psychiatrist seeing a depressed woman at this time of life is likely to suggest treatment with HRT rather than an antidepressant medication. Some researchers now believe that low mood is due to sleep disturbance – especially lack of REM sleep – linked with falling oestrogen levels or brought on by other menopausal problems such as night sweats and insomnia.

Symptoms of mild depression can include:

- nervousness
- anxiety
- agitation
- tiredness during the day
- exhaustion
- headache
- loss of self-esteem

- lack of confidence
- comfort eating
- weight gain
- low mood
- feeling sad
- crying for no apparent reason.

Symptoms of a more serious depression include:

- lethargy and listlessness with loss of interest in life
- loss of concentration
- continual weepiness for no obvious reason
- feeling slowed up both physically and mentally
- loss of sex drive
- difficulty sleeping
- early morning waking (between 2 and 5 a.m.)
- loss of appetite with weight loss
- feelings of worthlessness
- feeling that life isn't worth living.

If you have any of the symptoms of more serious depression, it is important to seek medical help before you get any worse. One in two cases of depression needing medical treatment remains undiagnosed, causing immeasurable sadness and despair.

The symptoms are due to an imbalance of chemical transmitters in the brain, which can be made worse by falling hormone levels. While in most cases the symptoms will eventually get better on their own, this can take months or even years. Drug treatment with antidepressants – which are not addictive – can boost levels of brain chemicals and help you start feeling better within a matter of days. In most cases, antidepressant tablets will need to be taken for at least 3–6 months before slowly stopping them. Alternatively, treatment with HRT may be suggested if this is thought to be your best bet (*see Chapter 7*).

Some women suffer from recurrent brief depression (RBD) around the time of the menopause. This is characterized by brief bouts of depression lasting 2 or 3 days, which suddenly lift. Low mood can strike up to 20 times per year and usually comes on suddenly. It is thought to be due to changes in brain activity and, as yet, there is no satisfactory drug treatment, although HRT is usually helpful.

Difficulty Concentrating and Poor Memory

Your memory is a personal storehouse of information. Around the time of the menopause, it is natural for your memory to become less like a filing cabinet and more like a sieve. You have three main types of memory:

1. Sensory memory – which stores information for only a split second
2. Short term memory – which stores facts for up to 5 minutes
3. Long term memory – which can store facts for as long as a lifetime.

Researchers are still unsure exactly how memory is stored, although one part of the brain in particular – the hippocampus – seems to be important in processing and storing long-term information. It is thought that new connections (synapses) are laid down between brain cells (neurones), and that new protein molecules are made to store information. It is possible that spare genetic material – DNA which is not being used to hold the genetic code – is involved, or that electrical circuits play a part.

Falling hormone levels affect your ability to store information for any length of time. It is worth developing a few tricks to improve your memory, such as writing notes to yourself on sticky pads and leaving them in obvious places. Supplements such as Ginkgo biloba, choline or lecithin can also help, as can using aromatherapy oils to boost your recall powers (*see Chapter 8*).

Food Cravings

Appetite, or the desire for food, is a very personal phenomenon. It is influenced by sensations of hunger but can produce insidious, niggling desires to eat even when your stomach is groaning with food.

Appetite is regulated by two areas in the brain – the *feeding centre* and the *satiety centre*. There is also a *thirst* centre regulating your intake of fluids. On top of this, the presence of food in certain parts of the gut also releases hormones that switch off your desire to eat.

Despite these regulations, some people can still eat through feelings of satiety because of especially strong appetite signals – or food cravings. These tend to become more common at times of hormone fluctuation, for example just before a period, and around the time of the menopause – probably due to the effects of hormone receptors in these parts of the brain.

When you eat carbohydrate, two things occur:

1. insulin is secreted by the pancreas
2. tiny amounts of a chemical called serotonin are released in the brain.

Both insulin and serotonin play a major role in controlling your eating behaviour and food choices. Insulin is a hormone that allows blood glucose to enter cells and provide a source of energy. Usually, just enough insulin is secreted after eating to cope with the exact amount of carbohydrate ingested. If you produce too much insulin, however, blood sugar levels may fall too quickly and you will experience food cravings, irritability and even feelings of faintness.

It is only when your insulin levels start to fall that release of serotonin is triggered in the brain. Serotonin is a neurotransmitter. It relays messages across important nerve connections (synapses) and has a number of different functions. These include influencing appetite, the way you select certain foods and the feeling of having eaten enough. Serotonin also gives you a chemical high that makes you feel good and can help to lift depression. Low levels of serotonin have been linked experimentally to over-eating and food cravings, and can occur around the time of the menopause.

Up to 50 per cent of women also suffer pre-menstrual syndrome (PMS) in which appetite is significantly increased and sugar (carbohydrate) is craved. This can result in eating over 500 extra calories per day. Over 80 per cent of women find they can help to control their food cravings by eating carbohydrate little and often. This also helps to lift your mood and may help to damp down annoying mood swings.

Following a wholefood diet with plenty of fresh fruit and vegetables and complex carbohydrates can help, as can avoiding table sugar as much as possible. When a snack attack occurs:

- Eat some carbohydrate such as a slice of wholemeal bread, a couple of plain crispbread or rice cakes – but avoid carbohydrate that come complete with extra fat such as a sausage roll, a cream cake or a doughnut.
- When you eat, chew slowly and pause between each mouthful so that the metabolic and emotional effects triggered by eating – and which tell you that you are full – have time to click in before you have eaten too much.
- If the craving continues, drink a glass of sparkling mineral water fortified with the juice of half a lemon, or try cleaning your teeth slowly with a strongly flavoured tingling toothpaste.
- Go for a brisk walk or take another energetic form of exercise.
- Eat a piece of fruit – a banana is a particularly good choice for satisfying your urge.

Chapter Four

THE MENOPAUSE AND YOUR SEX LIFE

Many women find that sex feels different after the menopause as a result of falling oestrogen levels. This can have both psychological and physical effects on your sex life. Not surprisingly, symptoms can lead to relationship difficulties, and many women become depressed. In most cases you will start to feel better as your body gets used to lower levels of oestrogen hormone.

Studies suggest that a third of women experience sexual difficulties around the menopause:

- 1 in 5 loses her sex drive altogether
- 1 in 5 suffers from vaginal dryness
- 1 in 6 develops difficulty in reaching orgasm
- 1 in 12 suffers from painful intercourse (dyspareunia).

These are all normal responses to falling oestrogen levels. If your symptoms are interfering with your life it is important to confide in your doctor – especially if you feel depressed. Don't be embarrassed – you would be surprised how often doctors deal with this sort of problem. You may find it helpful to take your partner along with you to the consultation. A loving, supportive partner is essential to get you through what can be a difficult time of life. In most cases, sexual difficulties can easily be put right – the important thing is to seek help, not let the problem build up until it causes major problems in your relationship.

VAGINAL DRYNESS

The most noticeable physical effect of lack of oestrogen is vaginal dryness. Every woman will notice this to some extent after the menopause unless she is taking hormone replacement therapy (HRT). Lack of lubrication means it is more difficult to become aroused and sex may be painful due to dryness. The clitoris also becomes less sensitive. In most cases, using a special water-based lubricant gel or pessaries such as *KY*, *Replens* or *Senselle* will help to revitalize a flagging sex life.

If the problem continues, it is important to see your doctor. There is a condition called Sjögren's Syndrome in which the eyes, mouth, nose, throat or vagina can start to dry up. This is linked with the immune system attacking the normal lubricating glands. Nine out of ten sufferers are women, mostly over the age of 30. If you have also noticed dry, gritty eyes, this condition is a possibility. It is not particularly serious, but you will probably need treatment with lubricants such as artificial tears for dry eyes or saliva for dry mouth.

CLITORAL HOOD RETRACTION

After the menopause, the tissues around your vagina naturally shrink and thin due to lack of oestrogen. In some women, the hood covering the clitoris becomes retracted. This exposes sensitive tissues full of nerve endings, which may make sexual stimulation intensely unpleasant. If this happens, don't be afraid to confide in your doctor. Oestrogen replacement, for example with cream or vaginal tablets, will quickly solve the problem.

LOSS OF SKIN SENSITIVITY

Unfortunately for women, the skin all over your body becomes less sensitive as oestrogen levels fall. One study found that 6 out of 10 post-menopausal women noticed skin numbness so that caresses from their partner were no longer enjoyable. Not surprisingly, nine out of ten of these women found this sensory loss interfered with their enjoyment of sex.

You may find that your skin sensitivity improves if your partner gives you a sensual massage. Use a ready-made sensual massage lotion or make one yourself by diluting one or more essential oils in a carrier such as Sweet Almond oil – use 15 drops essential oil per 30 ml carrier oil. (For more on aromatherapy, *see Chapter 8*.)

You may also find that taking an Evening Primrose Oil supplement and following a diet rich in plant hormones helps. In most cases, HRT will also quickly bring skin sensitivity back up to normal.

DIFFICULTY REACHING ORGASM

One in six menopausal women finds it more and more difficult to reach orgasm. This is probably due to lowered sensitivity of the clitoris as oestrogen levels fall.

Normally, during female sexual arousal fluid is secreted into the vagina to provide lubrication. The upper third of the vagina lengthens and expands, becoming very sensitive to touch. The entrance to the vagina becomes swollen and tighter to grip the penis more firmly. During orgasm, nerve impulses spread through various nerves to cause contraction of pelvic floor muscles and sometimes of your thigh muscles as well.

When oestrogen levels are low, however, vaginal lubrication is scant. Because your vaginal tissues are also starting to shrink, expansion of the upper vagina and tightening of the lower vagina may not occur. There are also changes in the way your nerves conduct electrical impulses, which means that orgasm is more difficult to achieve, and that when it does occur the sensation is less intense – this is also linked to weakening of pelvic floor muscles in women who have previously had several children, or large babies (*see* Stress Incontinence, *page 69*). You may also notice leaking of urine during orgasm.

A study in which ultrasound probes recorded what happened during intercourse in women found that when the male penetrated a woman from behind or the side, she achieved a better orgasm than in the 'missionary' position. It is worth trying different positions until you find one that suits you best.

LOSS OF SEX DRIVE

Loss of sex drive is the most common sexual problem to affect women, especially after the menopause. Your sex drive is controlled by the interaction of the female hormones oestrogen and progesterone, plus the male hormone, testosterone. The level of testosterone in women is much lower than that in men and varies widely. Women who have higher levels of active testosterone tend to have a higher sex drive. Testosterone in women is mainly produced by the ovaries, so after the menopause testosterone levels usually fall, although small amounts of testosterone-like hormones (androgens) are also made by:

- the adrenal glands
- the skin
- muscle cells
- the brain and pineal gland
- hair follicles
- body fat stores.

During the menopause, these other androgen sources take over testosterone production from the ovaries and their output of androgen hormones double. In some women, this is so successful that their sex drive may even increase as the effects of testosterone become more pronounced without oestrogen to counter-balance them. This is also one reason why you may start to develop unwanted, coarser hairs on your chin and upper lip.

If you have been under long-term stress, however, your adrenal glands may have no extra reserves to take over some of the hormone-producing functions of the ovaries.

Research shows that sexual interest falls off more rapidly in women than men between the ages of 50 to 60 years. By the age of 70, half of all women admit to having little interest in sex, compared with only 10 per cent of men at the same age. According to a recent survey, women aged 20–29 make love around 5 times per month, while women aged 55–59 make love twice a month or less. Half of all women in the 55–59 age group reported not having sex at all in the previous month.

Although it is difficult to talk about embarrassing problems such as these, it is important to talk to your partner. Any frequency of making love is normal so long as both of you are happy about it. Many couples share love, affection and a meaningful emotional relationship without a physically active sex life. Frequently, however, particularly where making love has virtually petered out, one of the partners will be unhappy about the lack of a physical relationship.

Loss of sex drive may not necessarily be due to the menopause. It is natural for sexual activity to decline the longer you have been in a relationship. You may need to work out why your desires have changed:

- Are there other problems in your relationship?
- Do you still find time to talk?
- Are you too tied up with work, running the home or caring for relatives?
- Do you and your partner still show affection for each other?
- Are you still friends?

If you still show affection towards each other and you still enjoy a cuddle together, lack of sex drive is unlikely to be due to one or other of you falling out of love, or to problems in your relationship. It may well be linked to your changing hormones, although it can also be linked with tiredness, anxiety, stress or illness.

- Make sure you get plenty of sleep – tiredness will quickly lower your libido.
- Avoid excessive stress – take regular time out for rest and relaxation.
- Take more exercise – this will boost your metabolic rate, improve your fitness level and burn off excess stress hormones – don't over do it, however.
- If you smoke, try to stop – research shows that smoking lowers hormone levels enough to bring the menopause

on up to 2 years earlier than normal, and will also affect your sex drive.
- Avoid drinking excessive amounts of alcohol. In the long term this can lower your sex drive, reduce vaginal secretions, shrink the ovaries and lead to menstrual problems. The intakes that trigger these problems vary from person to person, depending on how your metabolism handles alcohol and how much exercise you take. Stick to the new safe maximum of up to 21 units alcohol per week for women.
- Take a good multinutrient supplement – lack of some vitamins and minerals, especially zinc, can cause hormonal imbalances and reduce your sex drive.
- Try also taking Evening Primrose Oil supplements – these contain essential fatty acids, which act as building-blocks for sex hormones.
- Check that a low sex drive is not an unwanted side-effect of any tablets you are taking – those that can affect your libido include drugs prescribed for high blood pressure, water retention, and depression.

Studies show that the quality of a woman's sex life gains significant benefits if she takes HRT:

- increased sexual frequency and enjoyment
- increased sexual fantasies
- increased vaginal lubrication
- decreased pain during intercourse.

HYSTERECTOMY AND YOUR SEX DRIVE

If your menopause has come on following a hysterectomy, you are more likely to notice changes in your sex life. When making love, the uterus moves upwards as you become aroused. During orgasm it contracts rhythmically to add to the intense sensations felt during climax. One in 3 women who have had a hysterectomy notices the loss of these uterine sensations when making love, and 7 out of 10 find it more difficult to achieve orgasm. Although there may be no difference in your sex drive at first, after a year women who have had a hysterectomy have significantly fewer orgasms per year than women with an intact womb. In a few cases, the opposite is true – some women find love-making more enjoyable and orgasm more intense after the operation, especially if they were previously in a lot of pain.

PAINFUL SEX

Deep pain during intercourse may be due to diseased ovaries, a prolapsed womb, or to the bladder or rectum bulging into the vagina to form a cystocoele or rectocoele. These problems often develop after the menopause, as lack of oestrogen allows pelvic tissues to thin and stretch.

If intercourse suddenly becomes painful for no obvious reason, it is important to tell your doctor. Both superficial and deep pain during intercourse have a variety of causes including a thrush infection, bacterial imbalance, endometriosis, an ovarian cyst or even an ectopic pregnancy. In most cases, the problem can be solved with proper investigation and treatment.

SEEKING HELP

If you have a sex problem that seems to be related to the menopause, it is best to seek help from your GP. If you have a physical problem such as vaginal dryness or painful intercourse, this needs to be investigated to make sure there is no infection or other problem present. Treatment with vaginal lubricants or HRT will often help to sort the situation out.

If you feel the sexual problem is linked to your relationship rather than the menopause, contact RELATE. Their local number will be in the telephone directory. Relate have a number of counsellors and sex therapists who are trained to help anyone cope with a relationship or sexual problem – sympathetically and in confidence.

Loss of sex drive which is not linked with other signs of oestrogen withdrawal such as thinning of vagina tissues may improve with combined oestrogen and testosterone therapy.

Testosterone is usually only prescribed to women by a doctor specializing in the area of menopausal problems.

Sensate Focusing

Sex therapists sometimes advise a form of treatment known as sensate focusing, or pleasuring, to help overcome lack of interest in sex. At first, penetrative sex is banned and the couple take turns to caress and explore each other during foreplay. You are encouraged to spend around an hour giving each other pleasure through massage, but avoiding obviously erotic areas such as the breasts and genitals. Once both partners are comfortable with this, you progress to the next stage: Genital Sensate Focusing, in which erogenous zones can be touched as well.

Mutual masturbation is allowed, but full intercourse remains out of bounds. This takes away any pressure to perform and allows the woman to relax without fearing intercourse. Eventually, sometimes after more than 20 sessions lasting an hour each, simple vaginal penetration without subsequent thrusting may be achieved. Later, penile thrusting is introduced as well.

Sex Positions to Try

Women-on-top positions help you to gain better control during love-making and can prove more satisfying for both of you. By moving up and down and varying the speed and depth of penetration, you can set your own pace so you are likely to reach orgasm more easily.

Penetration from behind can give you a more satisfying orgasm, as this thins and stretches the front wall of the vagina where the 'G spot' is said to be situated. Lean forward from the hips, either while standing up or when kneeling on a bed or armchair. Support yourself by holding onto the headboard or back of a chair. Your partner should penetrate you gently from behind while holding on to your waist or buttocks. Another position good for stimulating the G-spot is to make love when lying curled up, side by side, your partner's front to your back (the 'spoons' position).

THE MENOPAUSE AND CONTRACEPTION

A woman in her forties is only half as fertile as a woman in her twenties, but still has a good chance of becoming pregnant. If you are having regular periods, this suggests that you are still producing an egg each month, even if you have started suffering from menopausal symptoms. If you have developed irregular periods and miss some monthly bleeds, this suggests that ovulation is not occurring during each cycle, but you must still consider yourself fertile. Many pregnancies occurring over the age of 40 are unplanned. Unless you would like to have a child at this time of life, it is important to use an effective method of contraception, as pregnancy in older women does carry additional health risks:

- the maternal mortality rate in the age group 40–49 is four times higher than for women aged 20–29
- the risk of a perinatal death for the baby is doubled as maternal age doubles (that is, there is twice the risk at age 40 as at 20, twice the risk at age 36 as at age 18, etc.)
- chromosome abnormalities in the foetus (such as Down's syndrome) are also more likely when the mother is over 35

If you do not wish to become pregnant, the best advice is to use a reliable method of contraception for at least 1 year after your last period – as long as this takes you past the age of 50. If you are still under 50, you should use contraception for a total of 2 years after your last period.

If you are taking HRT, you may still be having regular monthly withdrawal bleeds. HRT is not a method of contraception – researchers in one study found that, out of 20 women aged 42–45 taking HRT, 12 (60 per cent) ovulated during the month they were assessed. If you are on HRT, you must use a reliable non-hormonal method of contraception (such as condoms, diaphragm) until your doctor advises that this is no longer necessary. HRT and hormonal methods of contraception are not usually given together (but *see* The Intra-uterine System, *page 66*).

Whatever method you use, you want to be confident that it is safe, effective, reliable and easy to use. Many women also want a method that is not too messy and which does not interfere too much with the spontaneity and pleasure of making love.

The aim of an effective method of contraception is to prevent fertilization through one or more actions, such as:

- acting as a physical barrier between sperm and egg
- affecting transport of sperm or egg through the female reproductive tract
- making the womb lining incompatible with pregnancy
- preventing ovulation.

A variety of methods of contraception are suitable for use around the time of the menopause. These are briefly reviewed below to help you decide which is right for you.

Method	Typical Failure Rates per 100 women (all ages) using method (per cent)
No Contraception	85
Natural fertility awareness	15
Male Condom	2–15
Female Condom	2–15
Diaphragm/cap	6–15
Coil (IUCD)	1–3
Progestogen Coil (IUS)	Less than 1
Combined Pill	1–8
Mini Pill	3–10
Depot Progestogen	Less than 1
Progestogen Implant	Less than 1
Female Sterilization	Less than 1
Male Sterilization	Less than 1
Morning-after Pill	1–4.

Natural Methods of Contraception

Withdrawal Method
The withdrawal method involves the male withdrawing from the female just before ejaculation. Withdrawal requires strong motivation, as the instinctive male reaction at orgasm is to thrust as far

forward as possible. Timing is important. If withdrawal occurs too early, orgasm will fail. If too late, semen will enter the vagina. Some sperm may also be released early along with the lubricating secretions from the Cowper's glands. Practised carefully, the withdrawal method can be surprisingly effective. Although there are many better methods of contraception available, withdrawal is better than nothing. It should not be relied on if it is imperative that pregnancy is avoided.

Fertility Awareness
Fertility awareness techniques are used to monitor a woman's body changes (such as temperature, position and texture of the cervix, changes in cervical mucus, breast sensitivity, etc.) to predict when ovulation has occurred. While this method can be effective, it can be less easy to assess changes in your cervix and cervical mucus during the menopause, especially if you suffer from vaginal dryness. A new method of contraception, Persona, uses a mini-computer and urine testing to measure hormone levels and assist fertility awareness.

Barrier Methods of Contraception

Male Condom
The male condom is made from vulcanized latex rubber – a polyurethane version is also available in some countries. This barrier method of contraception is useful around the time of the menopause. It offers good protection with careful use and, as each condom should be used with additional spermicidal cream or gel, it provides additional lubrication. Make sure you only use a water-based lubricant, as petroleum jelly, mineral oils such as baby oil – and even some HRT vaginal cream preparations – weaken latex and can reduce condom strength by up to 95 per cent within 15 minutes. The most reliable condoms are those certified with the European CE mark or the British Standard Kitemark.

The Female Condom
The female condom is a pre-lubricated, disposable, polyurethane sheath that fits loosely inside the vagina. It contains two flexible

rings – a smaller, inner ring which sits loosely inside the sheath and holds the condom in position beyond your pubic bone, and a larger ring, attached to the rim, which remains outside your body. The female condom is as effective as the male condom, and over a hundred times less likely to burst during use. The female condom is a useful method of contraception during your menopausal years as it lines your vagina, providing the equivalent of a second skin. This is especially useful if you suffer from dryness or superficial discomfort or tenderness during sex.

The Vaginal Diaphragm

The diaphragm is a dome-shaped device made from latex rubber. It varies in size from 50–100 mm in diameter and needs to be tailor-made for you by a trained family planning specialist. After insertion, the diaphragm is designed to cover the cervix and upper vagina, stopping sperm from entering your upper reproductive tract. The diaphragm is kept in place by a firm spring or hinge within its rim plus the action of your vaginal muscles and pubic bone. A diaphragm should always be used with a water-based spermicidal gel or cream – your vagina naturally balloons upwards during sexual arousal, which may make it possible for some sperm to pass between the side of the device and the upper vaginal wall if spermicide is not used. The spermicide has the added advantage of providing extra lubrication. You will need to have the diaphragm fit rechecked if your weight fluctuates (up or down) by more than 2–3 kg (half a stone).

Hormonal Methods of Contraception

Modern hormonal methods of contraception can usually be continued right up until the menopause, unless you have a medical reason for not taking them. Women who smoke are usually advised to stop taking the combined oral contraceptive Pill (COCP) at the age of 35, as smoking and the COCP together significantly increase the risk of developing a blood clot.

Because hormonal contraceptives contain artificial hormones – usually different ones from those found in HRT – they can mask menopausal symptoms. Some women therefore find that when they stop using a hormonal method of contraception in later life, their periods suddenly stop or they suddenly develop menopausal symptoms.

Hormonal methods of contraception are not usually given together with HRT.

The Combined Oral Contraceptive Pill (COCP)

The combined oral contraceptive Pill is one of the most reliable methods of contraception, so long as you remember to take it correctly. It contains 2 synthetic hormones, an oestrogen and a progestogen. It is taken every day for 21 days, and then a 7-day Pill-free interval occurs during which a progestogen withdrawal bleed usually occurs – you are still covered against pregnancy during this 7-day break. The combined Pill works by:

- inhibiting secretion of Follicle Stimulating Hormone and Leutinizing Hormone in the pituitary gland so that egg follicles fail to mature each month and ovulation stops
- thickening cervical mucus so sperm cannot swim through easily
- slowing transportation of sperm and eggs in the Fallopian tubes
- thinning the lining of the womb so that if an egg does become fertilized, it cannot implant or develop.

As long as there are no other medical reasons for stopping taking it, you can continue using the COCP right up until the end of your fertile life, should you choose to.

The COCP is highly effective against unwanted pregnancy, but is associated with a number of side-effects. While most women tolerate the COCP very well, possible side-effects include:

- weight gain
- nausea
- headaches
- breast soreness
- bloating
- changes in sex drive
- mood changes
- intolerance to contact lenses

- breakthrough bleeding
- changes in vaginal discharge – with more or less produced
- high blood pressure
- increased risk of blood clots – especially in smokers
- jaundice
- possible increased risk of breast cancer.

The Pill also has some beneficial effects on health. It protects against cancer of the ovaries or womb and reduces the risk of pelvic inflammatory disease (PID), benign breast disease and of some ovarian cysts. It also makes your periods regular, reduces monthly blood loss and can help to prevent pre-menstrual syndrome.

WHAT TO DO IF YOU FORGET TO TAKE A COCP

For maximum contraceptive protection, it is important to avoid lengthening the 7-day Pill-free interval. This means it is worse to miss pills at the beginning or end of the pack rather than those in the middle – contrary to popular belief. During the Pill-free week some ovarian follicles may start to develop, but they will disappear once you start taking the next pack of pills. Any pills missed on either side of the Pill-free break may allow follicle development to progress to the point of ovulation, however.

If you forget to take a COCP but remember before it is 12 hours overdue, take it immediately and then take the next Pill as normal when it is due. If you forget to take the COCP and only remember when it is more than 12 hours late:

- Take it immediately and take the next Pill when it is normally due – even if this means taking two Pills close together.
- Use extra precautions (such as condoms) for the next 7 days.
- Count how many Pills are left in the pack after the Pill you've forgotten to take. If **7 or more** Pills remain, leave the usual break after this pack before starting the next pack. If **less than 7** Pills remain, start a new pack the day AFTER finishing this one – that is, don't have the usual 7-day break.

If two or more Pills have been missed, especially from the first five at the start of a packet, you should consult your doctor about whether it is worth taking emergency contraception (the morning-after Pill).

Gastro-enteritis (diarrhoea and vomiting) will interfere with absorption of the COCP; if you are suffering from this you should use an additional method of contraception (such as condoms) if you make love, during your illness and for 1 week after.

The Progestogen-only (Mini) Pill

The progestogen-only Pill (POP) contains a single synthetic hormone, a progestogen, in a much lower dose than that in the COCP. It is useful for women who cannot take oestrogen hormones, for women over the age of 35 who smoke, and for women who wish to come off the COCP or stop using the contraceptive coil towards the end of their fertile lives. The POP works by:

- thickening cervical mucus so sperm cannot swim through
- thinning the endometrial lining of the womb so if an egg is fertilized, it cannot implant or develop
- decreasing motility of sperm and eggs within the Fallopian tubes.

It does not necessarily stop ovulation – in around 60 per cent of cycles, eggs are still released, although the effects described above make pregnancy unlikely, especially as the menopause approaches.

The progestogen-only Pill is usually started on the first day of a period – you are then protected against pregnancy within about 4 hours. The POP is taken consecutively every day without a tablet-free break (even during menstruation) and must be taken within 3 hours of its due time to be effective. If delayed, cervical mucus starts to liquefy and contraceptive protection may be lost. Most menstrual bleeds occurring while taking the mini-Pill are light and regular, every 28 days.

As the POP contains only one hormone and in a much lower dosage than that found in the COCP, it is associated with fewer side-effects. There is no evidence of an increased risk of cancer, blood clots or high blood pressures. The main side-effects are to do with periods, which may become irregular or disappear altogether.

Some studies suggest that it is linked with an increased risk of ectopic pregnancy.

The mini-Pill produces its main effect on cervical mucus thickness within 4 hours of being swallowed. This effect slowly wears off during the next 24 hours. Even if a mini-Pill is only 3 hours late (that is, 27 hours since the last tablet) you should use extra precautions whenever you make love during the next 7 days.

If two or more Pills have been missed, emergency contraception should be considered.

Gastro-enteritis will interfere with absorption; additional contraception should be used during the illness and for 1 week after.

Progestogen Injection

The contraceptive injection (depot progestogen) is a slow-release store (depot) of a synthetic progestogen hormone which is injected into your buttock (or arm) during the first 5 days of your menstrual cycle. Depending on the injection used, it needs to be repeated every 8 or 12 weeks.

The injection works in the same way as the mini-Pill but is more effective as it stops ovulation in most cycles. As the injection is a slow-release preparation, its effects can last for longer than expected and a return to fertility may be delayed for several months – even up to a year or longer from the date of the last injection. It is an ideal method of contraception for a woman approaching the menopause, whose family is complete, and who prefers not to have to remember to take a contraceptive pill each day.

Minor side-effects are common and mostly linked to a woman's period pattern – half of all women stop having periods while receiving the injections.

Depot progestogen has no serious side-effects and may protect against PID and cancer of the womb. (Long-term use of depot progestogen, however, may increase your risk of osteoporosis; *see Chapter 5*.)

Progestogen Implants

The progestogen implant consists of 6 flexible tubes filled with a slow-release, synthetic progestogen hormone. The 6 capsules are implanted in a fan shape on the inside of your upper arm under local anaesthetic. Ideally, they should be inserted on the first day of a period; they will then protect you against pregnancy within 24 hours.

The implants work in the same way as the mini-Pill, by thickening cervical mucus, thinning the womb lining and reducing motility of eggs and sperm within the Fallopian tubes. Release of an egg still occurs in around half of all menstrual cycles. Once implanted, the method provides contraceptive cover for up to 5 years, after which the capsules must be removed and replaced if the method is to be continued. This may be a suitable method of contraception for women approaching the menopause, assuming that you can expect to have up to 5 years of fertile life ahead of you. It is less ideal for women whose periods are likely to stop naturally within the next year or two.

The most common side-effects are increased bleeding and spotting during the first 3 months of use, which occurs in a third of women. Another third stop having periods altogether. Most menstrual changes settle down over the next 7 to 9 months. Other side-effects are similar to those occurring with all hormonal methods of contraception, for example headache, depression, mood changes and weight gain.

There have been some difficulties reported with removal of the implants. Make sure your doctor is experienced in removing them: ask how many he or she has removed, and how many have been a problem.

Another hormonal method of contraception – the intra-uterine system (IUS) – is now also available. It is a cross between a progestogen implant and the coil – *see page 66*.

Intra-uterine Devices

Intra-uterine Contraceptive Device

The IUCD (sometimes also known as the coil) is made from polyethylene and copper, and placed inside the womb cavity to prevent pregnancy. Two monofilament threads hang down into the vagina to help with future removal and to let you check that the device is still in place.

The IUCD prevents pregnancy in a number of ways:

■ It triggers a low-grade inflammation in the womb lining, making it inhospitable to a fertilized egg and interfering with transportation of sperm and egg within the Fallopian tubes.
■ The copper ions are toxic to eggs and spermatozoa.
■ It physically interferes with implantation of a fertilized egg.

The main side-effect of the coil is the production of heavier, more painful periods, which can even cause iron-deficiency anaemia. Some women also experience bleeding or spotting between periods. IUCDs are also linked with an increased risk of PID and ectopic pregnancy. Although the IUCD is a possible method of contraception to choose in the years approaching the menopause, it is probably best reserved for women who have already been using it for some time. The intra-uterine system (*see below*) is much preferable at this time of life.

The Intra-uterine System (IUS)

The intra-uterine system (IUS) is a new and unique method of contraception. It delivers a synthetic progestogen hormone (similar to that found in the progestogen-only mini-Pill, depot injection and progestogen implant) directly into the uterus via a coil-like device made of plastic which is surrounded by a sleeve of hormone which is slowly released into the uterus. It remains effective for up to 5 years before needing to be replaced. The amount of hormone that reaches the bloodstream is so low that it is equivalent to taking only 2 progestogen mini-Pills per week.

The IUS prevents pregnancy by:

■ suppressing the normal function of the womb lining (endometrium) so that a fertilized egg cannot implant
■ thickening cervical mucus to prevent sperm getting through
■ interfering with development of ovarian follicles – although it does not stop ovulation altogether.

The IUS is as effective as female sterilization, but has the advantage of being reversible. It is also free from many of the side-effects associated with the IUCD and other progestogen methods of contraception. The most common side-effect is a change in your normal bleeding pattern. Your first 3 periods may last longer than normal, and you may notice some spotting between periods. After this, your periods will become lighter and for many women blood loss dwindles to almost nothing each month. One in five women stop having periods altogether – a welcome event in most cases. The IUS also relieves painful periods and there seems to be no increased risk of PID or ectopic pregnancy. A few women notice hormone-related effects for the first few weeks, which may include headache, breast tenderness, skin problems or nausea, but these are uncommon.

The IUS is currently under trial as a new method of delivering HRT. The progestogen hormone is delivered via the IUS as normal, while the oestrogen tablets are taken by mouth. This makes the IUS ideal as a method of contraception for women who also need oestrogen replacement therapy for menopausal symptoms or for protection against increased risk of osteoporosis or coronary heart disease. If the trials are successful, this treatment may become routine in the near future.

Sterilization

Sterilization is an ideal option if your family is complete and you still have several years of potentially fertile life ahead of you. Many couples choose vasectomy rather than female sterilization, as the operation is less invasive and can be performed under local anaesthetic.

Vasectomy

Vasectomy can be performed under a local or general anaesthetic. Two sperm-carrying ducts, the vas deferens, are cut and tied (or sealed by heat) through a small incision in the scrotum. The operation usually takes 10–15 minutes. Complications are rare, but can include bleeding, swelling, bruising and infection.

It takes around 3 months for sperm already in the storage ducts to disappear from the semen, and an alternative method of contraception must be used until the man is told his ejaculate is free of sperm. Around 1 in 2,000 vasectomies subsequently fails when the tubes rejoin spontaneously.

Female Sterilization

There are two ways of performing female sterilization under a general anaesthetic:

1. Slim women with no previous abdominal problems can usually undergo a laparoscopic (keyhole) sterilization that takes 15–20 minutes. Two small incisions are made – one in the navel and one in the pubic hair line. Gas is pumped into your abdominal cavity to push your bowel out of the way, then a viewing instrument (laparoscope) is inserted and the Fallopian tubes identified.
2. Larger women, or those who have abdominal adhesions (perhaps as a result of previous surgery or abdominal infection), or those in whom laparoscopic sterilization proves difficult for whatever reason are sterilized during an open operation (mini-laparotomy). A 5-cm long incision is made along your bikini line to expose the womb and Fallopian tubes.

The Fallopian tubes may be closed by the application of special clips, cut and tied, or cut and the ends sealed by heat. A relatively new procedure involves passing an instrument (hysteroscope) into the womb through the vagina and plugging the exits where the Fallopian tubes join the womb from the inside, but this is not yet widely available.

Unlike male vasectomy, female sterilization provides immediate protection against pregnancy. While it is an option for women approaching the menopause, a reversible method of contraception may be preferable if you only have a few fertile years ahead of you, as all operations carry a small but significant risk of complications or after-effects.

Chapter Five

THE MENOPAUSE AND STRESS INCONTINENCE, OSTEOPOROSIS, AND HEART DISEASE

THE MENOPAUSE AND STRESS INCONTINENCE

Stress incontinence – the leakage of urine due to physical exertion (stress) such as coughing, sneezing or even just walking – is thought to affect at least 60 per cent of menopausal women. Some cases are mild, resulting in only slight damping, but a few women are devastated by a total loss of bladder control. Unfortunately, half of all sufferers never consult their doctor either through embarrassment or a mistaken belief that nothing can be done. In fact, 7 out of 10 cases of stress incontinence are curable with the right treatment.

Stress incontinence is due to weakness of the pelvic floor muscles so that the neck of the bladder is no longer properly supported, allowing it to sag. This causes the opening around the urethra (tube through which urine flows from the bladder to the outside) to open. Sometimes, the bladder also bulges into the front of the vagina, causing a pouching known as a cystocoele. Most cases are linked with childbirth, especially if you have had large babies or many children. This stretches the pelvic floor muscles, which at first causes few problems. It is only after the menopause, when oestrogen levels fall and tissues start to thin, that the weakness shows up.

Lack of pelvic floor support places strain on sphincters keeping the bladder and urethral openings closed. A sudden increase in intra-abdominal pressure as happens during lifting, coughing, laughing, sneezing or running then results in urine leaking out. Many sufferers cut down on their fluid intake in an attempt to combat the problem, but this in fact only makes matters worse:

Your urine becomes concentrated, more irritant and is also more likely to produce a detectable smell. Even if you have problems with leaking urine, it is important to maintain an adequate fluid intake of at least 2–3 litres a day.

When you consult your doctor, a urine sample will be analysed to rule out any infection (cystitis) and you will be gently examined to assess your pelvic organs and look for any prolapse (that is, loosened pelvic organs that have bulged or come down out of their usual site). In some cases, further investigation is needed to measure your urinary flow, bladder pressure, and to see whether your bladder muscles are irritated. If you have pure stress incontinence, however, you will usually be referred to a physiotherapist or incontinence advisor to learn pelvic floor exercises – these produce a dramatic improvement in 30–70 per cent of women.

If you are able to take hormone replacement therapy (HRT), this will help to return your tissues to their pre-menopausal state and to cure mild cases of incontinence, as well as increasing the chance of success with exercises or surgery. If HRT tablets or patches aren't suitable for you, you may benefit from the oestrogen vaginal ring or oestrogen vaginal tablets, which sit in place in the vagina and supply oestrogen locally to tissues with little being absorbed into the circulation (*see page 114*). The older oestrogen creams are less acceptable as they are messy and some hormone is absorbed into the bloodstream, which is not always desirable; many women soon stop using them.

Pelvic Floor Exercises

Pelvic floor exercises aim to strengthen and build up the muscles supporting your bladder and urethra so that leakage of urine no longer occurs. There are two types of muscle fibre involved:

1. slow-twitch fibres – which need multiple repeated contractions to retrain them
2. fast-twitch fibres – which need maximum 'squeeze' effort to retrain them.

Once you have been taught the exercises to do, you will need to practise them several times a day, little and often – some contractions will be quick short ones, while others will last up to 10 seconds. These exercises can be done virtually anywhere and are undetectable to anyone else.

Simple exercises include:

- pulling up your front and back passages tightly as if trying to stop your bowels and bladder from opening. Hold tight for a count of 4; repeat this every hour, increasing in frequency as you find them easier to do.
- When on the loo, practise stopping the flow of urine midstream. Initially this will be difficult, but when it becomes easier try to do it at least once a day to maintain improvement.
- Some women find it difficult to identify the muscles involved – in which case you may be shown how to insert one or two fingers into your vagina so that you can practise squeezing these until you can recognize which muscles are involved.

To test the strength of your pelvic floor muscles, once a month try jumping, running or skipping on the spot to see if you leak any urine. You will be advised to repeat these exercises regularly throughout the day (such as in 10 sets of 10) and should start to notice an improvement within 3 months. Continued progress should follow over several months. It is important to persevere – exercising at regular intervals every day – as progress can be slow (though sure). If you seem to reach a point where no further improvement occurs, however, consult your doctor for further advice.

Other tips to improve stress incontinence include:

- Pull in your pelvic floor muscles before coughing, sneezing or lifting
- Avoid standing for long periods of time.
- Lose any excess weight, which puts unwanted extra pressure on pelvic floor muscles
- Eat plenty of fibre and drink plenty of fluids to avoid constipation – straining to open your bowels will weaken your pelvic muscles
- Avoid carrying heavy weights

- Make sure your bladder is completely empty after each visit to the bathroom
- Take regular exercise to tone up muscles throughout your body.

Other Treatments

If pelvic floor exercises alone have not solved the problem, a number of other measures can help:

- Physiotherapists can strengthen your pelvic floor muscles using a tiny electric current – two electric pads are placed on the perineum (tissue between the vagina and anus) to stimulate the muscles at regular intervals.
- You can be given tiny weighted cones to wear inside the vagina for 10–15 minutes twice a day – weights vary from 5 g to 60 g. This will help to tighten and tone your muscles, which have to contract to hold the cones in place.
- A new urethral balloon device can be fitted into the neck of the bladder. The balloon in the tip is then inflated to block urine leakage – it is designed for you to use yourself after 20 minutes' training, and comes with reusable applicator.

Collagen Injections

A new treatment is now available for stress incontinence, which involves injecting collagen around the urethra and neck of the bladder under local anaesthetic – usually two injections are given, one on either side of the urethra. The collagen increases tissue bulk at the neck of the bladder and helps to keep the opening of the bladder closed. Before the collagen is injected around your bladder, you will need to have a small injection of collagen into your skin to make sure you are not allergic to the preparation. Studies show that over 80 per cent of women notice a marked improvement, with 60 per cent becoming totally dry. Less than 4 per cent of women notice little or no benefit. Two years on, almost 70 per cent of women treated still reported improvement, with 50 per cent completely dry. Most women need to have the bladder collagen implants repeated at occasional intervals, as the collagen is slowly absorbed into the body.

Surgery for Stress Incontinence

Traditional surgery for improving stress incontinence has a 95 per cent success rate. It involves stitching a nylon sling under the neck of the bladder to provide support, tightening loose tissues and sometimes taking in vaginal tucks (colporrhaphy) if the bladder or rectum are prolapsing through the vaginal walls. This tightens the vagina as well as helping to support the bladder and, as a bonus, many women find this also improves their sex life.

Sometimes, prolapse of the uterus makes it difficult to correct stress incontinence unless the womb is removed. If your family is complete, a vaginal hysterectomy may be the best option. This can be performed at the same time as surgery to support the neck of the bladder and – as the womb is removed through the vagina – has the advantage of not leaving an abdominal scar.

THE MENOPAUSE AND OSTEOPOROSIS

Osteoporosis – one of the most common conditions to affect post-menopausal women – has reached almost epidemic proportions in the Western world. This is despite the fact that it is largely a preventable disease. In the UK, for example:

- Over 3 million people suffer from osteoporosis.
- Osteoporosis affects 25 per cent of women by the age of 60.
- Osteoporosis affects 50 per cent of women by the age of 70.
- One in 4 women develops an osteoporotic fracture during her life.
- Every 3 minutes, someone suffers an osteoporotic fracture.
- 40 people die every day as a result of an osteoporotic fracture.
- More women die from hip fracture than from cancer of the ovary, cervix and uterus combined.

Women are relatively protected against osteoporosis until they reach the menopause. This is because the female hormone, oestrogen, acts on bone to increase its mineral content. Once oestrogen levels fall after the menopause, bone thinning naturally occurs.

While strong bones are to a certain extent inherited, diet and lifestyle – especially during childhood and adolescence – is important to build up strong, thick bones before you reach the menopause and they start to thin. Obviously, the stronger your bones are, the less likely you are to reach a stage where your bones have thinned down enough for fractures to occur. If bone density is even 10 per cent below the average value for a young, otherwise healthy woman, her risk of osteoporosis in later life is more than doubled.

What Is Osteoporosis?

Bone is a living tissue containing a network of collagen fibres filled with calcium salts. Bone is constantly remodelling itself, with as much as 10 per cent of its mass broken down and rebuilt each year – your entire skeleton is replaced every 7–10 years. This remodelling process involves special cells (osteoclasts) dissolving old bone, while other cells (osteoblasts) lay down new bone.

The osteocytes and osteoblasts put out fine finger-like projections that interconnect and communicate with each another. This network seems to be sensitive to the everyday stresses and strains on each bone, and can indicate exactly where a bone needs building up. Researchers do not know exactly how the process of bone remodelling is started and stopped, although various hormones and growth factors are known to be involved.

In osteoporosis, the balance between bone production and bone absorption is distorted, so that the amount of both collagen fibres and calcium salts falls significantly. This makes bones thin and brittle so they fracture more easily. Osteoporotic bones may have so few minerals in them that they show up as pale ghosts on x-ray rather than as strong white shadows.

There are two sorts of bone in your skeleton:

1. dense, cortical bone which forms a strong outer shell around each bone
2. cancellous (trabecular) bone forming the spongy, central filling of each bone.

Cortical bone is heaviest and accounts for 80 per cent of the skeletal weight. Because it is so dense, it is replaced quite slowly. Cancellous bone makes up only 20 per cent of skeletal mass but, because it is less dense, it is reabsorbed more quickly. Over half of all osteoporotic fractures occur in the less dense, cancellous bone.

The Symptoms of Osteoporosis

Osteoporosis has been described as a silent epidemic, for there are few symptoms or signs, even when the disease is advanced. Unfortunately, the first indication that you have a problem is usually when a fracture occurs after a minor fall. Fractures of bones in the spinal column (vertebrae) can occur spontaneously or result from minor strains when lifting or even coughing. These vertebral fractures are usually painful and can lead to a stooped posture and loss of height. In women, this pronounced spinal curvature is sometimes referred to as 'Dowager's hump'.

Recent evidence suggests that early osteoporosis may cause back pain – at least in men. Spanish rheumatologists looked at 81 men with osteoporosis (average age 55) and found that in 85 per cent of cases, back pain was the first symptom. Of these, 65 per cent suffered from long-term back pain. In half the cases, this was due to a previous vertebral fracture, but most men also had a history of back pain not due to fracture.

Who Gets Osteoporosis?

Although osteoporosis is often thought of as a disease of old age, it can affect anyone – even young women and children. People who are at most risk of osteoporosis are those who:

■ have a strong family history of the disease
■ are underweight

- have suffered from anorexia or bulimia nervosa in the past
- eat a calcium-poor diet, for example women on a continual slimming diet, or those who eat few dairy products
- are pregnant or breastfeeding and have a calcium-poor diet
- smoke or drink heavily
- take little exercise
- exercise excessively, such as marathon runners, ballet dancers and exercise trainers.

One in three hip and vertebral fractures occurs in men, but in four out of five cases there is an underlying problem such as underactive testes (hypogonadism) – the male equivalent of the female menopause – or a history of taking oral corticosteroids or drinking heavily.

What Causes Osteoporosis?

Loss of calcium from the bones is a normal part of the ageing process. Some as yet unknown signal triggers an increase in the number of bone reabsorbing cells (osteoclasts), so that more bone is absorbed than is rebuilt by the bone-building cells (osteoblasts). This leads to loss of collagen fibres and calcium salts so that bones become increasingly brittle.

- Bone density is lost most rapidly in the 10 years after the menopause once oestrogen levels fall.
- The average post-menopausal woman loses 2–3 per cent of her bone mass each year.
- Some lose as much as 5 per cent of bone density each year.
- By the age of 70, the bones of many women weigh 30 per cent less than before the menopause – in a few they may weigh a staggering 50 per cent less.

Women who are most at risk of osteoporosis are those entering the menopause early, before the age of 45 – especially if this was due to hysterectomy and surgical removal of the ovaries – and who have not taken HRT.

If your bone mass is already low by the time you reach the menopause (as, for example, because you have inherited thin bones, or because of a calcium-poor diet), your risk of a fracture is doubled. The rate at which you lose bone after the menopause is also important. Some post-menopausal women lose bone very quickly, due to an inherited tendency, a calcium-poor diet or immobility. If you have thinner bones than average when you reach the menopause, then continue losing bone mass at a faster than normal rate, your risk of suffering from an osteoporotic bone fracture is more than trebled.

MAIN RISK FACTORS FOR DEVELOPING OSTEOPOROSIS

- early menopause (under 45 years of age)
- regular use of oral corticosteroids for 3 months or longer
- hysterectomy, especially if accompanied by removal of both ovaries
- loss of periods (amenorrhoea) for any cause except pregnancy
- (excessive dieting, excessive exercise, use of depot progestogen contraception)
- excessive weight loss or being significantly underweight
- close family history of osteoporosis
- history of prolonged bed rest, especially in childhood
- heavy smoking
- being housebound with little exposure to sunlight and low dietary
- intakes of vitamin D and calcium
- liver disease
- overactive parathyroid glands (hyperparathyroidism).

How Osteoporosis Is Diagnosed

Osteoporosis may not be diagnosed until you have an x-ray to investigate a fracture after a minor fall. If the condition is suspected, however, you may be offered bone mineral density screening to assess how strong your bones are. Technology with impressive-sounding names such as Duel Energy X-ray Absorptiometry (DEXA) or dual photon absorptiometry (DPA) can accurately measure bone mineral density in the sites most prone to fracture – the femoral head (hip) and lumbar vertebrae (spine).

Bone density screening cannot accurately predict who will go on to have a fracture in later life if not treated. Two thirds of fractures occur among women whose bone density level does not fall below the lowest 20 per cent, which limits the effectiveness of global screening. As osteoporosis is a preventable disease, it is important to take steps as early as possible to safeguard your bones.

Preventing Osteoporosis

It is never too late – or too early – to take steps to reduce your risk of osteoporosis. This means:

- following a balanced diet providing adequate supplies of calcium and other important nutrients (such as magnesium, trace elements, zinc) essential for bone health
- getting enough vitamin D (from diet and exposure to sunlight)
- taking regular exercise
- stopping smoking
- avoiding excessive intakes of alcohol
- maintaining your fitness, balance, alertness and eyesight as you get older to minimize the risk of falls
- using walking aids when necessary, thinking ahead about safety in the home
- avoiding medications that may lead to confusion, dizziness or falls.

Calcium

Your body contains around 1.2 kg calcium stored in the skeleton, while around 10 g is dissolved in your body fluids.

- 99 per cent of calcium absorbed from the gut goes straight into your bones and teeth.
- 1 per cent plays an important role in blood clotting, muscle contraction, nerve conduction, regulating metabolic enzymes, energy production and the smooth functioning of the immune system.

Dietary calcium is absorbed in your small intestine, a process that is dependent upon the presence of vitamin D. The process is not that efficient: usually only 30–40 per cent of dietary calcium is absorbed from the gut; the remainder is lost in your bowel motions.

How Much Calcium Do You Need?
The National Osteoporosis Society recommends the following daily intakes of calcium:

children 1–12 years	800 mg per day
teenagers 13–19 years	1,200 mg per day
pregnant and breastfeeding teenagers	1,500 mg per day
women 20–40 years	1,000 mg per day
pregnant and breastfeeding women	1,200 mg per day
men 20–60 years	1,000 mg per day
women over 45 on HRT	1,000 mg per day
women over 45 years not on HRT	1,500 mg per day
men and women over 60 years	1,200 mg per day

In 1990, the average calcium intake in the UK was 820 mg per day.

Diet

A balanced diet containing good supplies of calcium-rich foods is essential for maintaining strong bones and to help prevent osteoporosis. Lack of dietary calcium means that your bone stores of calcium are raided to maintain normal blood calcium levels. If this continues for any length of time, your risk of future osteoporosis is significantly increased. Good intakes of calcium are therefore vital throughout life – during childhood and adolescence when bones are still developing, as well as in later years when bones are naturally starting to thin down. Low intakes of calcium have also been linked with an increased risk of high blood pressure and stroke. In fact, drugs that promote calcium channels in the body are highly successful in treating hypertension, angina, some irregular heart rhythms and poor circulation.

Dietary sources of calcium include:

- milk – semi-skimmed and skimmed milks actually contain slightly more calcium than full-fat and are better for your overall health
- dairy products such as cheese, yoghurt, fromage frais
- green leafy vegetables such as broccoli
- salmon, especially tinned
- nuts and seeds
- pulses
- white and brown bread – in the UK, white and brown flour (but not wholemeal flour) are fortified with calcium by law
- eggs.

Some types of dietary fibre (phytates from wheat in unleavened bread, such as chapatti) can bind calcium in the bowel to form an insoluble salt that you cannot absorb.

CALCIUM CONTENT OF SOME FOODS

Food	Calcium Content
skimmed milk (600 ml)	720 mg
semi-skimmed milk (600 ml)	720 mg
whole milk (600 ml)	690 mg
soya milk (600 ml)	78 mg
whole-milk yoghurt (150 ml)	300 mg
low-fat yoghurt (150 ml)	285 mg
cheddar cheese (30 g)	216 mg
fromage frais (30 g)	27 mg
cottage cheese (30 g)	22 mg
2 slices white bread	76 mg
2 slices brown bread	76 mg
2 slices wholemeal bread	41 mg
1 egg	25 mg
1 large orange	58 mg
spinach, boiled (112 g)	672 mg
broccoli (100 g)	56 mg
winter cabbage, boiled (112 g)	43 mg
sardines (56 g)	220 mg
salmon, fresh (100 g)	29 mg
salmon, canned (100 g)	93 mg
Brazil nuts (56 g)	101 mg

| figs, dried (28 g) | 78 mg |
| baked beans (112 g) | 50 mg |

People on long-term slimming diets – especially crash ones – and those suffering from anorexia nervosa obtain little in the way of calcium-rich foods. Severe dieting also encourages excessive loss of calcium in the urine. If food intake is restricted so much that menstruation stops, oestrogen levels fall and bone thinning becomes rapid.

SYMPTOMS OF POSSIBLE CALCIUM DEFICIENCY:

- muscle aches and pains/twitching and spasm/cramps
- tetany (sustained cramps)
- palpitations
- receding gums/infected gums (periodontal disease)
- loose teeth.

Boosting Calcium Absorption from the Gut
In order to process dietary calcium, you need a good supply of vitamin D. This is made in small amounts in the skin on exposure to sunlight. It is also present in fish liver oil, oily fish (such as sardines, mackerel, herring, tuna, salmon, pilchards), eggs, liver and fortified milk or margarine (which must contain vitamin D by UK law).

As well as a calcium-rich diet, a high intake of fruit and vegetables has recently been shown to protect against osteoporosis. These foods contain micronutrients such as potassium, magnesium and vitamin C which are important for bone health.

A diet rich in essential fatty acids (EFAs) seems to stimulate uptake of calcium from the gut, to lower calcium loss in the urine and to trigger increased laying down of calcium in your bones. The EFAs of most benefit are those found in Evening Primrose Oil and oily fish. Good sources of EFAs include:

- sunflower and rapeseed oils
- evening primrose oil
- most nut oils (except peanut)
- dark green leafy vegetables

- oily fish – such as mackerel, herring, salmon, tuna and sardines.

Should You Take Calcium Supplements?

Ideally, as much calcium as possible should come from your diet. The easiest way to boost your intake is to drink an extra pint of skimmed or semi-skimmed milk per day, which will provide an extra 700 mg daily of calcium. If you are unable to tolerate dairy products, however, calcium supplements are important. Some supplements contain calcium salts which are relatively insoluble and pass through the gut unabsorbed. For this reason, effervescent tablets, or those that dissolve in water to make citrus-flavoured drinks are thought to be better. New formulations free of sodium, potassium and colour are also available. People with a tendency to kidney stones should only take calcium supplements under the supervision of a doctor.

Research suggests that adding calcium supplements to the diet of elderly people reduces their risk of a vertebral fracture by 20 per cent, while giving them both calcium and vitamin D supplements reduces their risk of non-vertebral and hip fracture by 30–40 per cent.

Factors Interfering with Calcium Absorption

Heavy consumption of alcohol, coffee, meat and salt can reduce the amount of calcium you absorb from your diet and are linked with low bone mass and early osteoporosis. Safe intakes of alcohol, however (up to 28 units per week for men, up to 21 units per week for women) may actually increase bone density and reduce the risk of osteoporosis, although this is still under investigation.

Long-term use of antacids containing aluminium have been shown to interfere with calcium deposition in bone, and if used regularly for more than 10 years can double your risk of developing a hip fracture.

Smoking cigarettes significantly increases the risk of osteoporosis. It lowers blood oestrogen levels and, as well as triggering a premature menopause up to 5 years earlier than normal, hastens bone thinning. By both stopping smoking and improving your diet, a woman can expect to delay her menopause by at least 3 or 4 years as well as reducing her future risk of osteoporosis.

Osteoporosis and Exercise

Regular exercise that is weight bearing and increases muscle strength is known to protect against osteoporosis by boosting the production of new bone. As well as stimulating blood circulation and increasing the supply of minerals to the bones, it also activates the bone network of cells (osteocytes and osteoblasts) to encourage strengthening in areas of high stress and weakness.

The types of exercise shown to have most benefit in stimulating bone regeneration are generally high impact (aerobics, gymnastics, netball, dancing, racquet sports, jogging, skipping). This type of exercise is most likely to appeal to younger, fitter people. Even walking, climbing stairs, carrying loads, doing housework and gardening have all been shown to protect against osteoporotic fractures. It is therefore important to maintain your level of physical activity in later life.

Try to do some exercise every day – a minimum of 20 minutes brisk exercise 3 times a week is recommended for optimum health. By strengthening your muscles and improving co-ordination, exercise also helps to reduce the likelihood of a fall.

Osteoporosis and HRT

By replenishing your falling oestrogen levels, HRT boosts formation of new bone and can prevent the rapid bone loss seen in the 10 years after the menopause. This protective effect continues for some years after HRT is stopped, but is not maintained indefinitely (*see Chapter 7*).

An exciting new class of drug may one day eradicate osteoporosis. Called selective estrogen (US spelling) receptor modulators (SERMs), they switch on oestrogen receptors in bone arteries and the heart but switch off those present in the breast and uterine tissues. This gives all the benefits of HRT without increasing the risk of hormone-dependent cancers.

The first of this class of drugs to be discovered (raloxifene) will soon be available.

THE MENOPAUSE AND WOMEN'S HEART DISEASE

Coronary heart disease (CHD) is often thought of as a male problem, yet:

- It kills more women each year than cancer of the cervix, uterus and ovaries combined.
- It accounts for the death of as many as 1 in 4 women.
- It results in the premature death (before the age of 70) of 1 in 15 women.

One advantage that women do have over men is that the female hormone, oestrogen, helps to protect against CHD until they reach the menopause. Once you reach the menopause, however, and your oestrogen levels fall, you lose this protective effect.

How Heart Disease Develops

The heart is made up of a special type of muscle (myocardium) which beats continuously and consumes a large amount of oxygen. It receives blood from two main vessels:

1. the left coronary artery
2. the right coronary artery.

CHD occurs when a coronary artery becomes narrowed or blocked – usually through a process of hardening and furring up called *atherosclerosis* – so that heart muscle no longer receives all the blood it needs. Tissue that is not receiving enough oxygen is said to be *ischaemic*; this triggers a type of heart pain known as angina – a tight pain behind the sternum that typically comes on during exercise and is relieved by rest. If oxygen supply is suddenly reduced (as by a clot blocking an artery) the ischaemic heart muscle cells suffer irreversible damage and some cells

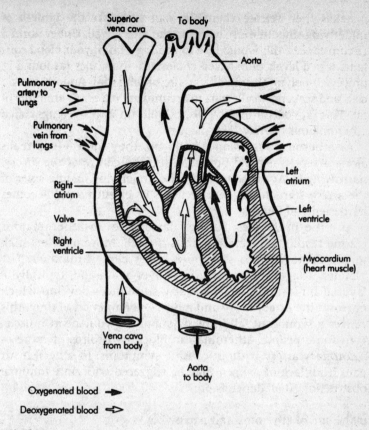

The heart

will die. Death of heart muscle tissue is known as a myocardial infarction or heart attack.

Atherosclerosis

The roots of atherosclerosis start early in life, usually in your teens. Normal wear and tear to blood vessel walls damages artery linings. Some of this damage is now thought to be triggered by inflammation, caused by certain fats in the diet. This damage is hastened by factors such as smoking cigarettes and high blood pressure. When damage occurs, small cell fragments (platelets) in the bloodstream stick to the arterial lining to form a tiny clot. The platelets then release chemicals that stimulate the growth of underlying smooth muscle cells in the artery wall. Under normal circumstances, this would lead to healing – but if your blood contains raised levels of oxidized cholesterol molecules (as found in processed polyunsaturated fats), the proliferating smooth muscle cells and scavenger cells start to accumulate excessive amounts of fat. This fat collects in the cells to build up into swellings called atheromatous (*porridge-like*) plaques.

As atheromatous plaques build up, they form fatty streaks along artery walls and protrude into the centre of the artery, narrowing it. At the same time, the underlying middle layer of the artery starts to degenerate, loses its elasticity and becomes hardened and fibrous.

As time progresses, further damage to an atheromatous plaque results in ulceration of its surface. More platelets stick to the damaged area to form a larger clot (thrombus). The platelets trigger the same process over again and, typically, a layered build-up of clot and fatty substances develop which narrows the artery more and more. Over a period of time, this causes a significant fall in blood supply to your heart muscle.

In some people, atheroma can block two-thirds or more of a coronary artery without causing symptoms. In others, heart pain from lack of oxygen may be triggered with only minimal obstruction. It all depends on:

- the site of atheroma and narrowing
- how good the blood supply from the other coronary artery is
- how well the two coronary arteries join up (anastomose) to share the load of supplying blood
- the type of coronary arteries you have inherited – wide ones like motorways or narrow ones resembling winding, country lanes.

In some cases, an atherosclerotic plaque eventually fractures, leading to haemorrhage within the blood vessel wall. This triggers a rapid build-up of thrombocytes to form a clot large enough to block the artery suddenly and cut off the blood supply to part of the heart muscle. This causes a heart attack (coronary thrombosis). The clot may also break off and wander around the bloodstream (thrombo-embolus) to impact else-where, commonly in the lungs or the brain.

Atherosclerosis can occur in arteries throughout your body – the only exception being your lungs. If widespread, hardening and furring of the arteries leads to high blood pressure, damage to internal organs (such as kidneys) and poor peripheral circula-tion (reduced blood supply to the legs). If the process impairs blood supply to the brain, gradual death of brain cells may lead to senility, while sudden blockage of a brain artery – or rupture of a damaged vessel – will cause a stroke.

Blood Cholesterol Levels

There are two sorts of cholesterol circulating in your blood-stream. One sort protects against CHD, the other seems to cause it. These fats (lipids) are transported around the body by carri-ers known as lipoproteins:

1. the harmful type is called LDL (low density lipoprotein) cholesterol
2. the beneficial type is called HDL (high density lipoprotein cholesterol.

The main difference between these two types of cholesterol is their size. LDL-cholesterol is a small molecule that can seep into dam-aged artery walls to fur them up. Scavenger cells (macrophages) can also engulf these molecules; as the macrophages try to leave the bloodstream to digest their meal, they become trapped in the arterial wall because they are over-laden with LDL-cholesterol molecules. This adds to the atherosclerosis process.

HDL-cholesterol, on the other hand, is a much larger mol-ecule. It is too large to be engulfed by macrophages, or to seep into damaged arterial walls, and stays in the bloodstream to do the work it is supposed to do. This includes carrying LDL-cholesterol around the body so that it is less likely to cause furring up and hardening of the arteries.

If you are told you have a raised blood cholesterol level, it is important to know whether your LDL- or HDL-cholesterol level is high:

- if your blood fats consist mainly of HDL-cholesterol, your risk of CHD is significantly reduced
- if most of the lipids are in the form of LDL-cholesterol, your risk of CHD is significantly increased.

You also have another type of fat in your blood, known as triglyceride. If your triglyceride levels are raised, your risk of CHD is also increased.

Classification of Total Blood Cholesterol Levels

Desirable	less than 5.2 mmol/l
Borderline	5.2–6.4 mmol/l
Abnormal	6.5–7.8 mmol/l
High	greater than 7.8 mmol/l

Studies suggest that 32 per cent of women in the UK have blood cholesterol levels that are above 6.5 mmol/l.

Normal Range for Various Blood Lipids

Total cholesterol	less than 5.2 mmol/l
LDL-cholesterol	less than 3.5 mmol/l
HDL-cholesterol	greater than 1 mmol/l
Triglycerides	less than 2.3 mmol/l

Slightly stricter criteria apply to men under the age of 30 and for those with CHD.

It is estimated that a rise in blood cholesterol of just 1 per cent increases your risk of CHD by 3 per cent. By reducing the average blood cholesterol level by 10 per cent, over a quarter of CHD deaths could be prevented.

HRT and Female CHD

Oestrogen also affects the way dietary fats are metabolized, raising blood levels of beneficial fats and lowering levels of harmful ones. Oestrogen also has an antioxidant effect (*see page 94*). Studies also show that taking oestrogen replacement therapy reduces the risk of CHD in post-menopausal women by up to 50 per cent (*see Chapter 7*).

The beneficial effects of HRT on blood fat levels is so striking that oestrogen is now considered by many doctors to be a cholesterol-lowering drug. In a trial involving post-menopausal women aged 40–60 years with high cholesterol levels, those receiving dietary advice plus HRT had blood LDL-cholesterol levels that were 19 per cent lower after 1 year – while women receiving dietary advice alone plus dummy HRT (placebo) only managed to lower their cholesterol levels by 5 per cent. The fall in LDL levels was less pronounced in overweight women and was greatest in non-smokers (20 per cent in non-smokers versus 2 per cent in overweight women). This trial suggests that HRT is an effective treatment for high blood cholesterol levels in post-menopausal women with an increased risk of CHD.

Another study showed that when over 800 women with severe coronary artery narrowing were given HRT, their risk of death from all causes was lower – after 10 years, 97 per cent taking HRT were still alive, compared with 60 per cent of similar women not receiving HRT. This protective effect was thought to be mostly due to a rise in the blood levels of protective HDL-cholesterol. Oestrogen has also been found to have a direct effect on blood vessel walls by:

- reducing damage to artery linings
- reducing the number of platelets that stick to the walls
- stabilizing atheroma plaques so they are less likely to trigger formation of blood clots
- reducing arterial spasm.

Syndrome X

Researchers have recently identified a problem that mainly affects menopausal women, which they have called Syndrome X. It is diagnosed if three features are present:

1. typical tight angina heart pain brought on by exercise
2. the heart muscle is shown to be lacking in oxygen when the patient is wired up to a heart monitor and exercises on a treadmill

3. no narrowing or blockages are found when the width of the coronary arteries is assessed using a special x-ray dye-test (angiography).

Further testing in these patients also rules out coronary artery spasm, high blood pressure, heart valve problems and other possible causes, which could possibly affect oxygen supply to the heart muscle.

At first, the cause of Syndrome X was a major puzzle. Then it was noticed that most patients affected were women, particularly post-menopausal women, with symptoms of oestrogen withdrawal such as hot flushes, nightsweats and headache. For example, out of 134 patients in one study, 27 were male and 104 were female, with an average age of 53.8 years. It also seems that women who have undergone hysterectomy are more prone to the condition.

Doctors now believe that Syndrome X is due to a hormone imbalance which affects the way small blood vessels (capillaries) in heart muscle react during exercise. Usually, they dilate to bring blood flooding into the exercising muscle. In Syndrome X, it is thought that these vessels fail to dilate so that the heart muscle lacks oxygen (becomes ischaemic) even though the coronary arteries are perfectly healthy.

While Syndrome X does not seem to be dangerous, in that it does not increase the risk of premature death, it does play havoc with people's lives: some patients are so intolerant of exercise they are virtually confined to their homes. Early studies show that giving oestrogen replacement therapy helps enormously by cutting down the number of angina attacks experienced and helping to relieve day-to-day symptoms.

CHD Risk Factors

Over 200 different risk factors have been linked with CHD, but not all of them are proven. For women, the risk factors that are most closely associated with atherosclerosis and having a heart attack include:

- increasing age after the menopause
- having a family history of CHD

- smoking cigarettes – cigarette smoking is directly responsible for 11 per cent of all female deaths from CHD
- having uncontrolled high blood pressure – 11 per cent of women are thought to be affected but are not receiving treatment
- eating a poor diet containing a high percentage of fat – especially saturated fat – and not enough fresh fruit and vegetables
- being overweight or obese
- having abnormally raised blood fat levels (cholesterol, triglycerides)
- not taking enough exercise
- drinking excessive amounts of alcohol
- having poorly controlled diabetes
- having high stress levels.

Modifiable Risk Factors

Although there is very little you can do to slow the ageing process or change the genes you have inherited, you can modify your lifestyle to reduce your risk of CHD. It is never too late to make these changes, even if you have reached the menopause and feel unhealthy. Your risk factors can be modified by:

- stopping smoking
- losing any excess weight
- exercising for at least 20 minutes, 3 times a week or more
- eating a healthy diet
- cutting back on salt intake to help reduce your blood pressure
- drinking no more than 2–3 units of alcohol per day
- avoiding excessive stress
- having regular check-ups to assess your blood pressure, cholesterol levels and general cardiovascular fitness
- considering taking HRT if you are eligible.

It is surprising what a difference these steps can make. Computer analysis of many trials suggests that for each risk factor you modify, your risk of CHD is lowered as follows:

Factor modified	Reduction in risk of CHD
Stopping smoking	50–70 per cent lower risk within 5 years
Losing excess weight	35–55 per cent lower risk for those who maintain a healthy weight
Exercise	45 per cent lower risk for those who exercise regularly
Reducing blood cholesterol levels through exercise, diet or medication	2–3 per cent lower risk for each 1 per cent reduction in blood cholesterol
Controlling high blood pressure	2–3 per cent lower risk for each 1 mmHg reduction of diastolic BP
Keeping alcohol intakes within healthy limits	25–45 per cent lower risk for those drinking at most 2–3 units per day
Taking HRT	44 per cent lower risk after the menopause
Taking prophylactic aspirin	33 per cent lower risk in users compared with non-users

The Benefits of Aspirin

Aspirin is a commonly used painkiller and anti-inflammatory drug that also has a powerful blood-thinning effect. It lowers the stickiness of platelet particles in the blood so that they are less likely to clump together and form unwanted clots. This effect occurs at only a quarter of the dose needed to relieve pain. Although there is not yet felt to be enough evidence to recommend that everyone takes prophylactic aspirin, it is surprising how many doctors take just half a tablet per day themselves for its considerable benefits. People who should consider taking a mini-dose of aspirin regularly every day include those who have:

- angina
- had a heart attack
- had a coronary artery bypass graft or dilation (angioplasty)
- had surgery for poor circulation in the limbs
- diabetes
- several major risk factors for CHD.

If you fall into any of the above groups and are not taking a junior aspirin per day, check with your doctor that it will suit you and fit in with any other medication that you are taking.

Studies suggest that prophylactic aspirin can reduce the risk of a first heart attack by 33 per cent in men – there is no equivalent data on its effects in women, but it is likely to be very similar.

Dietary Changes for a Healthy Heart

People who follow a Mediterranean-style diet have a 75 per cent lower risk of CHD than those eating a typical Western diet. The Mediterranean way of eating is thought to reduce the risk of atherosclerosis because it provides plenty of garlic, olive oil, antioxidant vitamins, oily fish and red wine, and is also rich in unrefined complex carbohydrates and fibre. These all help to keep your blood pressure, blood cholesterol levels and artery linings healthy.

Garlic
Garlic has been shown to have powerful protective effects against CHD. Scientific research has shown that it can:

- lower blood pressure enough to reduce the risk of a stroke by up to 40 per cent
- reduce the risk of CHD by up to 25 per cent
- lower harmful LDL-cholesterol by 12 per cent
- lower triglycerides by 13 per cent
- improve circulation by 48 per cent, especially through small blood vessels (as in the skin)
- lower the risk of blood clots by decreasing blood stickiness and platelet clumping
- hasten the breakdown of any clots that do form
- help to prevent dangerous heart rhythms.

The main substance derived from garlic is called allicin. Allicin is made from the interaction of enzymes and chemicals stored in uncut garlic cloves. Once the garlic is bruised or cut, these chemicals mix together to trigger production of the powerful smelling allicin.

Olive Oil
Olive oil is rich in a type of fat (oleic acid) that is monounsaturated. This is processed in the body to reduce blood levels of the harmful LDL-cholesterol without affecting your levels of desirable HDL-cholesterol.

Antioxidant Vitamins
Antioxidants help to protect your tissues, artery linings and your body fats – including the cholesterol in your bloodstream – from oxidation. Oxidation is a side-effect of harmful chemicals (free radicals) produced as a by-product of your metabolism. Dietary antioxidants help to mop up these free radicals before they can do any damage. The most important dietary antioxidants are vitamins C, E and betacarotene, and the mineral selenium. Good dietary sources of these dietary antioxidants include:

Betacarotene	carrots, sweet potatoes, sweet corn, spinach, broccoli, red or yellow peppers, parsley, watercress, spring greens, tomatoes, cantaloupe melons, apricots, peaches, mangoes
Vitamin C	blackcurrants, guavas, kiwi fruit, citrus fruit, mangoes, green peppers, strawberries, broccoli, sprouts, watercress, parsley, potatoes
Vitamin E	wheatgerm oil, avocados, broccoli, wholemeal cereals, nuts and seeds, oily fish

Oily Fish
Oily fish such as salmon, trout, mackerel, tuna and sardines contain an essential fatty acid known as EPA (eicosapentanoic acid). This is processed in your body to reduce blood stickiness, platelet clumping and the formation of unwanted blood clots. Eating oily fish can lower your risk of CHD and, if a heart attack should occur, lowers your risk of dying from it. A diet rich in oily fish (or fish oil supplements) can also help to prevent a second heart attack.

Red Wine
Over 20 studies around the world have shown that a moderate intake of alcohol reduces the risk of CHD by up to 40 per cent. In

particular, drinking wine – especially red wine – seems to be more beneficial than drinking beer or spirits. Red wine contains antioxidants; if taken with food, it neutralizes the effects of saturated fats in the diet. Surprisingly, people who drink small to moderate amounts of alcohol have a lower risk of CHD than teetotallers – though of course excessive drinking can increase your risk of a heart attack. Alcohol intake should be limited to 2–3 units per day for women.

Fibre

Eating the equivalent of 30 g fibre per day will decrease your risk of CHD, as dietary fibre absorbs fats in the gut. This means the fats reach your bloodstream more slowly, so that your body can handle them more easily. The most beneficial type of fibre seems to be soluble oat fibre – just 3 g per day (roughly equivalent to two large bowls of porridge) can lower total blood cholesterol levels by up to 0.16 mm/l. This is a small, but significant change.

Healthy Diet

If you want to reduce your risk of CHD, the following dietary guidelines are recommended:

- Eat a wholefood diet with as few processed and pre-packed foods as possible.
- Increase your intake of complex carbohydrates (wholegrain cereals, brown rice, wholemeal pasta, wholegrain bread) so that they provide at least half your daily energy intake.
- Eat at least 5 servings of fresh fruit, salad or vegetables every day (for example, a glass of unsweetened orange juice with breakfast, a large salad at lunch, 2 pieces of fruit during the day plus 2 veg with your evening meal).
- Cut back on your intake of fat, especially saturated fat. Switch to low-fat products and use more olive oil (or rapeseed oil), which have beneficial effects on blood cholesterol levels.
- Cut back on the amount of red meat you eat – eat more fish and vegetarian meals instead, including pulses and beans for protein. When you do have meat, buy lean cuts and trim all visible fat and skin.

- Increase the amount of fish – especially oily fish – that you eat, aiming for at least 300 g (2–3 servings) per week.
- Increase the amount of pulses, nuts and seeds you eat to an average of at least 30 g per day – they provide essential fatty acids which have beneficial effects on blood cholesterol (walnuts are especially good for you).
- Avoid sugary, fatty snacks.
- Cut back on salt intake – avoid salty foods such as crisps, bacon, tinned/cured/smoked/pickled foods; do not add salt to food during cooking or at the table; obtain flavour from herbs, spices and black pepper instead.

  Consider taking daily food supplements:
  - vitamin C (60–300 mg or more), vitamin E (10–50 mg or more), beta-carotene (6–15 mg)
  - standardized garlic tablets (600–900 mg)
  - omega-3 fish oil capsules.

Additional ways to lower your intakes of dietary saturated fat:

- Replace butter and cream with monounsaturated products derived from olive oil or rapeseed oil.
- Switch to low-fat brands of mayonnaise, salad dressing, cheese, milk, yoghurt etc.
- Have regular vegetarian days – but don't over-indulge in hard cheese or eggs.
- Avoid foods high in saturated fat such as coconut, creamy soups, chocolate, pâté, oysters, prawns.
- Cut down on cakes, chips, biscuits and crisps.
- Grill food rather than frying.
- Eat baked potatoes rather than roasted or chipped.

Chapter Six

STRESS AND THE MENOPAUSE

If you are under stress this can have a profound effect on the type of menopause you experience. Women who lead a demanding, stressful life seem more likely to suffer distressing menopausal symptoms, and this is now thought to be due to the lack of adrenal gland reserves, which normally provide some back-up to the failing ovaries.

Usually, up to 5 per cent of circulating sex hormones are made by your adrenal glands. As your ovaries stop working, your adrenal glands take over some of their function and produce small amounts of oestrogen as well as doubling their output of testosterone-like male hormones (androgens). If you have been under long-term stress, however, your adrenal glands may already be working flat out producing stress hormones such as adrenaline. When your menopause approaches, they have no extra reserves to boost their output of sex hormones.

WHAT IS STRESS?

Stress is a modern term used to describe the symptoms produced when you are under excessive pressure. A certain amount of stress is necessary to meet life's challenges, but too much is harmful and can leave you feeling tired, angry and tense. The symptoms of stress result from high levels of circulating adrenaline hormone which are secreted to prepare your body for conflict or escape. Adrenaline puts your systems onto 'red alert' so that your:

- blood sugar levels rise to provide energy
- bowels empty (nervous diarrhoea) so you are lighter for running – some people may also vomit if their stomach is full
- pupils dilate so you can see better
- pulse and blood pressure increase significantly
- breathing deepens (hyperventilation) so more oxygen reaches your muscles
- circulation to some parts of the body (such as the gut) shuts down, so more blood can be diverted to muscles.

In primitive days, these effects helped survival by preparing a person to face up to or flee from danger. Nowadays, the effects of stress build up inside you rather than getting burned off through a sudden burst of physical activity. Your body stays on 'red alert', leading to stress-related problems and panic attacks.

PHYSICAL SYMPTOMS OF STRESS

- tiredness
- sweating
- flushing
- nausea
- insomnia
- palpitations
- rapid pulse
- dizziness
- faintness
- trembling
- pins and needles
- numbness
- headache
- chest pain
- stomach pain
- diarrhoea
- period problems.

EMOTIONAL SYMPTOMS OF STRESS

- loss of concentration
- inability to make decisions
- a tendency to become vague and forgetful
- over-defensiveness and inability to take criticism
- extreme anger
- overwhelming feelings of anxiety and panic
- fear of rejection
- fear of failure
- feelings of guilt and shame
- negative thoughts
- moodiness
- loss of sex drive/sexual problems
- obsessive or compulsive behaviour
- feelings of isolation
- a feeling of impending doom.

A lot of these symptoms are similar to those that occur as a result of the menopause, and it can be difficult to untangle whether your problems are hormonal or stress-related. As menopausal symptoms in themselves can lead to stress, it is worth trying relaxation and breathing exercises to see if these help.

BREATHING EXERCISES

Breathing is an unconscious action which you rarely think about. Stress will quickly change your breathing pattern so that you over-breathe or hyperventilate with quick, irregular, shallow breaths. This occurs when your fight-or-flight mode is triggered but not completed. As a result, you inhale too much oxygen and exhale too much carbon dioxide, causing an imbalance of gases in the lungs. This makes the blood too alkaline, leading to dizziness, faintness and a sensation of 'pins and needles' in the face and limbs. This in turn creates panic and a cycle of anxiety – hyperventilation is set up.

Fast, shallow breathing sends messages to the brain that you are under stress and keeps the body on 'red alert'. Habitual hyperventilators may also experience chest pains, palpitations, sleep disturbances and other physical symptoms. Research has suggested that chronic anxiety can be caused by hyperventilation rather than hyperventilation being a symptom of anxiety itself.

Use the following exercises to control your breathing in situations where you feel stressed. They only take about 2 minutes and nobody around you will notice.

WHEN FEELING GENERALLY TENSE

- Sit back.
- Move your arms so that your shoulders are drawn back and down.
- Expand your chest and take a deep breath, filling your lungs as much as possible.
- Breathe in and out as deeply as you can, being aware of the rise and fall of your abdomen – not your chest. Repeat 5 times. Don't hold the breath in, just breathe naturally but more deeply than usual.
- Continue to breathe regularly, getting your rhythm right by counting '1, 2, 3' when breathing in and '1, 2, 3, 4' as you exhale.

WHEN PANIC RISES

- Say 'STOP' quietly to yourself.
- Breathe out deeply, then breathe in slowly.
- Hold this breath for a count of 3 and breathe out gently, letting the tension go.
- Continue to breathe regularly, imagining a candle in front of your face. As you breathe the flame should flicker but not go out.
- Continue breathing gently. Consciously try to relax – let your tense muscles unwind and try to speak and move more slowly.

Stretching Exercises to Relieve Stress

Try the following when you need a quick break or as general energizer:

ARM SWINGING

- Stand up and take a few deep breaths.
- Stretch both arms in front of you at shoulder height.
- Let your arms relax and drop to your sides, allowing them to swing to a natural standstill. Repeat several times.
- Finally, raise your arms above your shoulders and swing them energetically.

HAND SHAKING

- Shake each hand and arm in turn for a minute or two.
- When you stop your muscles will feel soft and relaxed.
- Repeat using your legs and feet if you wish.

RELAXING YOUR NECK

- Imagine you are carrying a heavy weight in each hand so that your shoulders are pulled towards the floor.
- 'Drop' this imaginary weight and feel the tension release. Repeat several times and feel your neck become less tense.

CIRCLING YOUR SHOULDERS

- Circle your left shoulder in a backward direction five times. Repeat with the right shoulder.
- Circle your left shoulder in a forward direction five times. Repeat with the right shoulder.
- Repeat, this time circling both shoulders at the same time.

General Relaxation

Have a bath or sit down quietly for an hour reading a book or magazine. Use an aromatherapy diffuser to fill the air with the scent of a relaxing essential oil (*see Chapter 8*). Have a candle-lit bath to which a diluted relaxing aromatherapy oil has been added.

Deep Relaxation

For a deep relaxation exercise which tenses and relaxes different muscle groups to relieve tension, set aside at least half an hour. This exercise is especially beneficial after a long soak in a warm bath.

Find somewhere quiet and warm to lie down. Remove your shoes and loosen any tight clothing. Close your eyes and keep them closed throughout the session.

First, lift your **forearms** into the air, bending them at the elbow. Clench your **fists** hard and concentrate on the tension in these muscles.

Breathe in deeply and slowly. As you breathe out, start to relax and let the tension in your arms drain away. Release your clenched fists and lower your arms gently down beside you. Feel the tension flow out of them until your fingers start to tingle. Your arms may start to feel like they don't belong to you. Keep breathing gently and slowly.

Now tense your **shoulders and neck**, shrugging your shoulders up as high as you can. Feel the tension in your head, shoulders, neck and chest. Hold it for a moment. Then, slowly let the tension flow away. Breathe gently and slowly as the tension flows away.

Now lift your **head** up and push it forwards. Feel the tension in your neck. Tighten all your **facial muscles**. Clench your teeth, frown and screw up your eyes. Feel the tension in your face, the tightness in your skin and jaw, the wrinkles on your brow. Hold this tension for a few seconds, then start to relax. Let go gradually, concentrating on each set of muscles as they relax. A feeling of warmth will spread across your head as the tension is released. Your head will feel heavy and very relaxed.

Continue in this way, working next on your **back** muscles (providing you don't have a back problem) by pulling your shoulders and head backwards and arching your back upwards. Hold this for a few moments before letting your weight sink comfortably down as you relax. Check your arms, head and neck are still relaxed too.

Pull in your **abdomen** as tightly as you can. Then, as you breathe out, slowly release and feel the tension drain away. Now blow out your stomach as if tensing against a blow. Hold this tension for a few moments, then slowly relax.

Make sure tension has not crept back into parts of your body you have already relaxed. Your upper body should feel heavy, calm and relaxed.

Now, concentrate on your **legs**. Pull your **toes** up towards you and feel the tightness down the front of your legs. Push your toes away from you and feel the tightness spread up your legs. Hold this for a few moments, then lift your legs into the air, either together or one at a time. Hold for a few moments and then lower your legs until they are at rest.

Relax your thighs, buttocks, calves and feet. Let them flop under their own weight and relax. Feel the tension flow down your legs and out through your toes. Feel your legs become heavy and relaxed. Your toes may tingle.

Your whole body should now feel very heavy and relaxed. Breathe calmly and slowly and feel all that tension drain away.

Imagine you are lying in a warm, sunny meadow with a stream bubbling gently beside you. Relax for at least 20 minutes, occasionally checking your body for tension.

In your own time, bring the session to a close.

EXERCISE AND STRESS

Regular exercise such as swimming, walking, cycling or other non-competitive sport will help you to overcome stress and make you more fit to cope with life's challenges. Adrenaline has primed you for activity; by exercising you will help to reverse its effects, burn off the stress hormones and reset your stress responses to a lower level. Try a non-competitive sport and spend at least 30 minutes exercising, 2 or 3 times per week – and put in enough effort to feel glowing and slightly out of breath. Even if you don't have time for regular exercise sessions, try to make activity part of your everyday routine, for example:

■ Walk part or all of the way to work.
■ Use the stairs rather than the lift wherever possible.
■ Do any household chores, such as hoovering, vigorously.
■ Swap watching television for a family bike ride or walk.

DIET AND STRESS

Caffeine and nicotine mimic the body's stress response and are best avoided when you are under pressure. Limit tea and coffee to 3 cups per day or switch to de-caffeinated brands. Take a good multinutrient supplement. Some vitamins and minerals such as vitamin C and the vitamin B complex are quickly used up during stress reactions. Vitamin B is further depleted by the metabolism of alcohol and sugary foods, often resorted to in difficult times. As vitamin B deficiency can in itself lead to symptoms of anxiety and irritability, a vicious circle is set in place.

■ Eat little and often to keep your blood sugar levels up – never skip a meal, especially not breakfast.
■ Eat a healthy, high-fibre diet full of whole foods.
■ Eat at least 5 servings of fresh fruit and vegetables every day.
■ Cut back on sugar, salt, saturated fats and processed or convenience foods.
■ Watch your alcohol intake and try to limit yourself to a maximum of 1 or 2 alcoholic drinks per day.

Chapter Seven

HORMONE REPLACEMENT THERAPY

HRT is one of the most beneficial developments in the area of women's health – for those who are able to take it. Current medical advice is that where HRT is indicated, it should ideally be prescribed until at least the age of 50 – and possibly for a further 8–10 years. This is particularly true for women who have had a hysterectomy and can take pure oestrogen replacement therapy. Computer simulations suggest that, taking all the risks and benefits into account, HRT is likely to prolong the life expectancy of a 50-year-old woman by up to a year. For a woman whose uterus is intact, and who needs to take combined oestrogen and progesterone replacement therapy the picture is less clear cut – having to take additional progestogen (a synthetic form of the female hormone, progesterone) may cancel out some of the beneficial effects of the oestrogen replacement itself.

Despite its benefits, HRT still remains controversial. It is linked with a number of side-effects, including a possible increased risk of breast cancer (*see page 121*). A surprisingly high percentage of women stop taking the treatment within a year of its being prescribed. In some cases this is due to genuine side-effects, but many women stop taking HRT without telling their doctor because of symptoms linked with the body's re-adjustment to the return of normal levels of circulating oestrogen.

Decisions about taking HRT involve very personal, subjective judgements. Some women regard the small increased risk of breast cancer as more significant than the reduction in the risk of heart disease. Others choose HRT in the hope of preventing an immobilizing hip fracture or painful osteoporotic collapse of their spinal vertebrae. Only you can decide whether you feel comfortable taking HRT, and for how long. The important thing is to have all the information at your fingertips so you can make an informed choice. This means questioning your doctor about the possible benefits and risks of HRT to you, bearing in mind your past medical history, lifestyle, inheritable family illnesses such as osteoporosis, heart disease or breast cancer, plus the effects of any other medications you are taking.

It is also important to keep in contact with your doctor so that if unwanted side-effects or unexpected problems do occur, you can discuss them and work out what is going on. Don't just stop taking HRT without telling your doctor first.

WHAT IS HRT?

HRT aims to give you back natural levels of the oestrogen hormone which your ovaries are no longer making. It may be prescribed for a number of reasons, including:

- to prevent a premature menopause in women whose ovaries have been removed
- the relief of menopausal symptoms such as hot flushes, night sweats and mood swings
- to treat vaginal dryness or stress incontinence
- to reduce your lifetime risk of coronary heart disease (CHD)
- to reduce your lifetime risk of osteoporosis
- possibly to reduce your risk of senile dementia.

The only hormone replacement needed is oestrogen – the other female hormone, progesterone, is thought to be less important from a health and symptom point of view. Unfortunately, however, oestrogen cannot be given on its own if you still have an intact uterus. This is because oestrogen alone will over-stimulate the womb lining (endometrium), making it plump up excessively. Over a period of time, this might result in abnormal cell changes (cystic hyperplasia) which have been linked with an increased risk of cancer of the womb. By giving progesterone as well during the last 10–14 days of the cycle, then stopping it, the endometrium is allowed to mature and shed. This mimics a period, but is more correctly known as a withdrawal bleed. As a result, HRT can protect against womb cancer.

If you have previously had a hysterectomy, you can be prescribed oestrogen-only HRT.

HRT AND MENSTRUATION

Until recently, for those women whose uterus was still intact and who therefore needed progesterone as well as oestrogen, taking HRT meant the return of a regular monthly bleed. Not surprisingly, this put a lot of women off HRT. New advances, however, mean that if you have not had a period for at least a year, taking HRT no longer has to mean the inevitable return of a monthly bleed:

- One synthetic hormone, called tibolone, has both oestrogen and progesterone effects in the body. This means it can control oestrogen withdrawal symptoms and protect the womb lining from over-stimulation without the need for separate progesterone. In 9 out of 10 cases it does not trigger the return of a withdrawal bleed as long as you haven't had a natural period for at least 1 year.
- Some new formulations of HRT provide continuous hormone therapy without triggering a monthly withdrawal bleed.
- One formulation provides a 70-tablet course of hormones, so that you only have a withdrawal bleed once every 3 months.

HRT VERSUS THE PILL

It is important to realize that HRT and the contraceptive Pill are very different:

- HRT restores oestrogen levels to the low normal blood range in women whose ovaries are no longer producing enough oestrogen. Overall, the total monthly dose you receive is less

than would normally be made by your ovaries in an average menstrual cycle.
- The contraceptive Pill, on the other hand, deliberately increases hormone levels above normal to approach those found in pregnancy. These high doses damp down the ovaries by fooling them into thinking you are pregnant so that no more eggs are released.
- The type of oestrogens used in the Pill are usually synthetic, while HRT tends to contain natural oestrogens which are identical to those found in the human body.

As a result, the risks and benefits of HRT are different from those of the contraceptive Pill. Oestrogens used in HRT are more natural, and less powerful, than synthetic oestrogens used in the oral contraceptive Pill. This means that HRT tends to have fewer side-effects and can also protect against osteoporosis and CHD. It is common for this to be forgotten, however – even by doctors. One study looked at 119 women newly referred to a menopause clinic because their GP thought contra-indications prevented them from taking HRT. In fact, none were felt by the consultants to have true contra-indications and all went on to receive HRT – many of the consultants felt that contra-indications such as a past history of high blood pressure or heart disease were in fact strong reasons why the women should receive the benefits of oestrogen therapy. Even patients with a previous history of breast cancer are now thought to benefit from HRT in some cases, as long-term follow-up studies suggest the benefits can outweigh the risks.

HRT AND MENOPAUSAL SYMPTOMS

Taking oestrogen replacement therapy quickly improves the symptoms of oestrogen withdrawal, such as:

- hot flushes
- night sweats
- difficulty sleeping
- vaginal dryness

- low sex drive
- bladder problems
- loss of skin sensitivity
- irritability
- mood swings
- anxiety
- tearfulness
- difficulty concentrating.

Some women opt to take HRT for 6 to 12 months to see them through this difficult period, then prefer to stop once their symptoms have passed or are more tolerable.

HRT, VAGINAL DRYNESS AND STRESS INCONTINENCE

Local oestrogen replacement with creams, pessaries, vaginal tablets or the vaginal ring (*see page 114*) will quickly improve symptoms of vaginal dryness and itching due to shrinkage of tissues after the menopause. If other symptoms are present, or if you need the additional benefits of protection against CHD or osteoporosis, systemic HRT taken by mouth will also treat vaginal or urinary symptoms.

HRT AND CORONARY HEART DISEASE (CHD)

Studies show that HRT reduces the risk of CHD in women past the menopause by up to 50 per cent. In women who have already had a heart attack, HRT provides 80 per cent protection against another one occurring. As a 50-year-old woman not on HRT has a 46 per cent chance of developing CHD and a 31 per cent chance of dying from it, the protection from HRT is significant. Oestrogen has this effect by lowering blood cholesterol levels (LDLs), by preserving arterial wall elasticity and by discouraging atherosclerosis (*see page 85*).

A 50-year-old woman has a 20 per cent chance of suffering a stroke during the remainder of her life and an 8 per cent chance of dying from one. Some studies show HRT has a beneficial effect on these figures, others don't. Overall, the effect of HRT on strokes is probably neutral.

HRT AND OSTEOPOROSIS

A 50-year-old woman has an overall 50 per cent chance of sustaining an osteoporotic bone fracture during the remainder of her life:

- a 15 per cent risk of hip fracture
- a 16 per cent risk of wrist fracture
- a 20–30 per cent risk of spinal deformity from vertebral collapse.
- and a 3 per cent chance of dying as a result.

Oestrogen slows bone loss and reduces the risk of developing a hip fracture by up to 40 per cent. Although bone loss continues once oestrogen therapy stops – and one study indicates protection against fractures is lost within 5 years of coming off HRT – treatment effectively buys your skeleton time. This means that bone thinning below the level linked with an increased risk of fracture is less likely to occur during your natural life span.

Interestingly, HRT seems to reduce the risk of an osteoporotic fracture more than would be expected from its effects on bone mass density alone. It may have other actions and increase the quality of new bone being made, as well as decreasing bone turnover.

HRT AND ALZHEIMER'S DISEASE

After the age of 65, the risk of dementia and Alzheimer's disease in women doubles every 4–5 years. By the age of 85, around 40 per cent of women suffer from dementia, especially among women who have previously had a heart attack (as these women are more likely to have hardening and furring up of arteries that affect the brain). As HRT helps to prevent CHD, it seems logical that it may also protect against dementia – especially as there are oestrogen receptors in the brain.

New research suggests that taking high-dose HRT decreases the risk of dementia or Alzheimer's Disease by 50 per cent; lower doses can still reduce the risk by as much as 40 per cent. This effect is most noticeable when HRT is used for more than 7 years. When oestrogen was given to 7 women with Alzheimer's disease, 6 showed a significant improvement compared with non-treated patients. It helped to improve memory, orientation in time and place, and their ability to work out simple sums. Improvement was noticed by carers, but the effect was lost when oestrogen was stopped. The addition of a progestogen (in this case, medroxyprogesterone acetate) appeared to wipe out much of the beneficial effects, however.

THE TYPES OF HRT PREPARATION AVAILABLE

New, improved formulations of HRT are becoming available all the time. Preparations available include:

- traditional tablets
- skin patches
- skin gels
- implants
- vaginal creams
- vaginal pessaries
- vaginal rings
- an intra-uterine progestogen coil used together with oral oestrogen tablets (currently under trial).

HRT taken by mouth is absorbed from the stomach into the bloodstream where it is taken straight to the liver along with nutrients absorbed from your food. Here, some of the oestrogen is broken down before reaching the rest of the circulation and oestrogen-sensitive tissues a few minutes later. As a result, doses given by mouth have to be larger than those delivered across the skin. In contrast, HRT absorbed through the skin (such as implants, patches, gels, creams, etc.) bypasses the liver and goes straight into the bloodstream, supplying your oestrogen-sensitive tissues before passing through the liver. This means the dose – and therefore the chance of side-effects such as nausea, is lower than with oral preparations.

As the heart pumps blood around your body, and HRT passes through the liver several times, it is slowly broken down and deactivated. Some is also passed out through the bile into your gut, where a percentage is reabsorbed to go around your system again. Oestrogen levels can therefore vary enormously from woman to woman at different times during the monthly cycle.

If any HRT preparation contains more than one formulation (such as two or more different coloured tablets containing a different blend of hormones per pack – or a patch plus a tablet), the pack will unfortunately mean a double prescription charge for those eligible to pay. Doctors tend to make up for this by prescribing 3–6 months' worth of HRT in one go once you are stabilized on a particular formulation.

Oral Tablets

If taking oestrogen-only HRT (that is, if you have had a hysterectomy) you take a tablet regularly every day without a pill-free break.

If taking a combined oestrogen and progestogen preparation, you will usually be prescribed a pack containing 21-, 28- or 91-day tablet courses. The progestogen will be given during the last 10–14 days of the cycle, either as a separate tablet or in a combined tablet which is a different colour to those at the beginning of the pack.

Some formulations give you a 7-day tablet-free break in which the withdrawal bleed occurs. In the majority of cases, you take tablets continuously – starting one 28-day course after another – and your period comes regularly while you are still taking tablets. With the newer 91-day formulation, you take tablets continuously but only have a bleed once every 3 months.

Skin Patches

HRT skin patches contain a hormone reservoir that is stuck onto the skin of the bottom, lower abdomen or hips and changed twice a week. A steady supply of oestrogen then crosses from the patch into the bloodstream, bypassing the liver to reach its target sites first. Most patches just contain oestrogen hormone, so if your uterus is intact you will need to take progesterone tablets for part of the cycle as well. One patch formulation has successfully managed to incorporate a progestogen into patch form – it contains 4 circular oestrogen only patches plus 4 larger, goggle-shaped patches in which each 'eye' contains either oestrogen or progestogen. The circular patches are used for the first half of your cycle, the goggle-shaped patches for the second half.

The patches can occasionally become dislodged and may release excess hormone in hot weather, or during vigorous exercise. Around 5 per cent of users develop slight skin irritation – this is minimized by applying each patch to a different part of your body than the previous one.

Skin Gels

Oestrogen gel is a cool, clear, colourless preparation that you squirt from a pressurized dispenser and rub onto the skin of your arm, shoulders or inner thigh. Two measures are used once a day – increased to 4 measures after a month if necessary. It is used on its own if you have had a hysterectomy. If your womb is still intact, you will also need to take progestogen tablets for 12 days of your cycle. Oestrogen gel is prescribed to relieve menopausal symptoms, vaginal dryness and the urinary problems linked with oestrogen withdrawal.

Implants

Oestrogen implants are small hormone reservoirs inserted under the skin of the lower abdomen using local anaesthetic and a special insertion device. This delivers a steady stream of oestrogen into the circulation, bypassing the liver to reach its target tissues first. Once it is inserted, it provides continuous oestrogen replacement for up to 6 months – if you have an intact uterus, you will need to take cyclical progestogen as well. Some evidence suggests that if too much oestrogen is released from the implant at first, this may trigger the return of hot flushes in some women when hormone levels fall again – even if levels are well into the normal range.

Vaginal Cream, Pessaries and Tablets

Oestrogen creams and pessaries can reduce vaginal dryness, help to reverse tissue shrinkage and increase vaginal lubrication. They sometimes also help with hot flushes, although absorption of oestrogen from the cream is not usually that great – they are prescribed in low doses to provide a local effect and so they don't over-stimulate the womb lining. The creams tend to be messy, are disliked by many women, and are only really suitable for short-term treatment. If prescribed long term, and if you have not had a hysterectomy, you may need to take an oral progestogen for 10–14 days each month.

Oestrogen creams are inserted into the vagina using a special applicator which you fill with cream yourself. At first you use the cream once or twice a day, then gradually reduce the frequency to 1–3 times a week. Every few months you will need to be re-examined and the dose may be reduced or discontinued as necessary depending on how well your tissues have responded.

Oestrogen pessaries are used by inserting 2 pessaries at night for 2–3 weeks only.

Oestrogen vaginal tablets are inserted with a special applicator – 1 tablet daily for 2 weeks, reduced to 1 tablet twice a week for 10 weeks. Treatment is then usually discontinued to assess your need for further treatment, and repeated as necessary.

NB: Many HRT cream formulations damage the latex of rubber condoms and diaphragms.

The Vaginal Ring

The vaginal ring is a convenient, non-messy way to deliver oestrogen hormone exactly where it is needed. Oestrogen reaches local vaginal tissues to improve lubrication but is not absorbed significantly into the bloodstream. It is therefore suitable for women who are unwilling or unable to take other forms of HRT. The vaginal ring needs to be removed or replaced every three months – either by a doctor or by the woman herself if she is happy to do this. The ring is left in continuously – even during menstruation and when making love (99 per cent of sexual partners are unable to detect it). At present this form of oestrogen can only be used continuously for two years, but the licence is expected to be changed so that the ring can be used for longer than this.

The Intra-uterine System

The intra-uterine system (IUS) is a hormone method of contraception similar to a coil that delivers a progestogen hormone (levonorgestrel) directly into the uterus. As a contraceptive it is as effective as female sterilization. It is free from many of the side-effects associated with the coil such as painful, heavy bleeding. Most women experience much lighter periods, and one in five women using the IUS will stop having periods altogether.

As the IUS delivers a continuous low dose of progestogen hormone, it is currently under trial in combination with oral oestrogen treatment for women needing HRT.

WHY WOMEN DON'T TAKE HRT

Up to 50 per cent of women are unable or unwilling to take HRT long term. Although many women start taking it, few continue long enough to receive its full benefits. Many women abandon HRT within the first few months – according to one study (in the US) the average time a woman took HRT was for 9 months; two-thirds of those starting treatment abandoned HRT within 1 year. Almost 60 per cent of post-menopausal women in the Western world have never taken HRT.

A recent survey of over 4,500 women found that the main reason for not using HRT was fear of side-effects. As a result, 45 per cent of women turned to alternative therapies – although only 27 per cent felt these remedies were beneficial.

When 752 women who had started and then stopped HRT were questioned, the following reasons for giving up treatment were given:

fear of side-effects	23 per cent
weight increase	13 per cent
no menopausal symptoms	15 per cent
physician's recommendation	13 per cent
bleeding disturbance	9 per cent
various non-specific reasons	27 per cent

Although 67 per cent said they would prefer a regime that did not produce withdrawal bleeds, only 9 per cent of HRT users claimed to have discontinued treatment because of bleeding problems.

Possible Side-effects of HRT

In most cases, the side-effects of HRT are minor, occur at the start of treatment, and settle down within a few weeks. Mild reactions are sometimes helped by changing the dosage or type of HRT. Some are more troublesome, however, so that treatment has to be stopped. They include:

- nausea and vomiting
- breast tenderness and enlargement
- breakthrough bleeding
- headache
- dizziness
- leg cramps or muscle pains
- increase in size of uterine fibroids
- intolerance to contact lenses
- skin reactions
- loss of scalp hair
- increase in body or facial hair
- pre-menstrual syndrome
- weight gain
- possible increased risk of breast cancer.

HRT should *not* be taken by women who:

- are pregnant or breastfeeding
- have had an oestrogen-dependent cancer (for example of the breast) unless their doctor agrees – an increasing number of experts now feel that women who have been successfully treated for cancer and have no evidence of a recurrence can take HRT
- have undiagnosed vaginal bleeding
- have active endometriosis
- have active blood-clotting disorders
- have severe heart, liver or kidney disease.

HRT should only be used with caution, and with careful monitoring by your doctor, if you have (or have a history of) any of the following conditions:

- migraine
- gall stones
- epilepsy
- diabetes
- high blood pressure
- fibroids of the womb
- a history of blood-clotting disorders
- mild on-going liver disease
- otosclerosis (a type of deafness)
- skin itching during a past pregnancy (pruritis)
- herpes gestationis (a rare blistering skin disease of pregnancy)
- multiple sclerosis
- porphyria (a rare metabolic disease)
- tetany (prolonged muscle spasm).

HRT should be stopped immediately and medical treatment sought if you become pregnant or develop:

- a first occurrence of migraine
- frequent, severe headaches
- sudden visual disturbances
- signs of a blood clot (such as thrombophlebitis,

thromboembolism) such as pain and swelling of a limb, poor circulation or discoloration of part of the body
- a rise in blood pressure
- jaundice.

While some doctors recommend that HRT is stopped 6 weeks before major planned surgery, others no longer feel this is necessary for normal, low-dose HRT – as long as heparin, a blood-thinning agent, is given after surgery.

CLONIDINE

HRT is not the only drug option for treating distressing menopausal symptoms. Menopausal flushing, recurrent headaches and migraine can also be helped by Clonidine, a non-hormonal drug that prevents dilation of the blood vessels. Clonidine is taken morning and evening and usually controls flushing and night sweats quite well. Possible side-effects include drowsiness, dry mouth, dizziness, nausea, constipation, sleeplessness and occasional rashes, although most women tolerate it well.

NATURAL PROGESTERONE

Natural progesterone is also gaining in popularity as a form of HRT. Unlike synthetic progesterone-like hormones (progestogens), natural progesterone cannot be given by mouth as it is quickly broken down in the gut – it must therefore be given as a suppository or topical cream to be absorbed into the circulation across a mucous membrane or the skin.

Progesterone usually has two main effects in the body:

1. It acts on the womb lining to increase its secretory functions, but only if the endometrium has been primed with oestrogen first.
2. It maintains pregnancy.

Research also suggests that progesterone has additional beneficial effects including protecting against cancer. Studies in the US suggest that women with normal progesterone levels are 5 times less likely to suffer breast cancer and 10 times less likely to suffer other forms of cancer compared to women with progesterone deficiency. Progesterone also seems to reverse some loss of bone density, improves hair loss and helps skin to retain its thickness and moisture levels.

Unfortunately, natural progesterone is often tarred with the same brush as synthetic progestogens which, because their chemical shape is different, have additional unwanted side-effects in the body. Unlike synthetic progestogens, however, natural progesterone:

- does not cause a fall in beneficial HDL-cholesterol levels or raise harmful LDL-cholesterol
- does not encourage fluid and salt retention in the body
- does not have virilizing effects and does not increase oiliness of skin or encourage unwanted hair
- does not cause breast tenderness, abdominal bloating or cramps
- does not cause pre-menstrual syndrome, anxiety, irritability or depression

In fact, natural progesterone has virtually no known ill-effects.

Some private physicians are prescribing progesterone creams for post-menopausal women unable to take oestrogen-containing HRT. There is logic behind this, as women who are not ovulating do not produce as much progesterone as those with a regular ovulatory cycle. Many researchers now believe that many women are in fact progesterone-deficient – especially if they have been on the Pill and exposed to synthetic progestogens for many years.

Doctors prescribing progesterone creams in the US have found that their patients have:

- increased their bone density
- had their hot flushes well controlled
- felt better in themselves with less anxiety or depression and improved energy levels

- suffered fewer aches and pains
- enjoyed a return of sexual appetite.

As yet, there are no long-term trials showing the benefits of progesterone in treating post-menopausal women. As a result, the Council of the British Menopause Society are concerned about the claims being made for natural progesterone products which have not been proven by properly controlled scientific studies. They state:

It has been well substantiated that oestrogen deficiency is a major factor in the development of menopausal symptoms, osteoporosis and cardiovascular disease in post-menopausal women. Properly controlled scientific trials reported in peer-review journals have confirmed the value of hormone replacement with naturally-occurring oestrogens ... We find claims for progesterone preparations particularly worrying. Although progesterone/progestogens may have some beneficial effects on hot flushes and bone density, there are not data provided on the amount of progesterone which is absorbed from these preparations.

Post-menopausal women should be reassured that [oestrogen] HRT remains the treatment of choice for menopausal symptoms, osteoporosis and cardiovascular disease and there is no scientific evidence to support a change to 'alternative' therapies ... The BMS has issued this statement in the hope that women will continue to seek informed advice from their medical practitioner or menopause clinic, and that those who are considering or currently taking HRT will not be easily dissuaded from obtaining the proven benefits of natural oestrogen replacement.

While oestrogen HRT should always be the first option considered for treatment of post-menopausal symptoms and for protection against CHD and osteoporosis, there are nevertheless some women who are unable to take it. For these women, natural progesterone products – and other alternative therapies – offer help and relief that they would otherwise be denied.

HRT AND BREAST CANCER

The thought of breast cancer is enough to strike fear in any woman's heart and, understandably for many, it is a stumbling block to taking HRT. HRT has been linked with an increased risk of breast cancer in some research trials, but not in others. Analysis of all the data has suggested that the relative risk of taking HRT may be as low as 1.07 times that of women not taking HRT, with this risk only increasing after you have taken HRT for 15 years. Results are not consistent, unfortunately, with some researchers suggesting that the relative risk may be significantly higher (1.32 times as great).

It is now thought that taking HRT may trigger breast cancer earlier in women who would have developed it anyway – but because of the screening that occurs when you are on HRT, and because the cancer is likely to be picked up earlier than would otherwise have been the case, there is no evidence that taking HRT increases your risk of *dying* from breast cancer. In fact, women who use HRT before developing breast cancer may have a lower risk of death from breast cancer, because stopping HRT will make a hormone-dependent tumour shrink. In addition, the health benefits in reducing risk of death from osteoporosis and CHD are indisputable.

One in 12 women will develop breast cancer in the UK – including at least 1 in 12 women who happen to be taking HRT. If you are taking HRT and do develop breast cancer, it will be difficult to believe that it is not connected to your treatment. It is therefore important to weigh up all the evidence carefully and decide with your doctor's help whether the benefits you are likely to get from HRT do offset any possible risks for you.

Breast Cancer – the Facts

In the UK:

- 1 in 12 women will eventually suffer from breast cancer.
- An average of 560 women are diagnosed each week.
- 26,000 women are newly diagnosed each year.
- Over 15,000 women die of breast cancer every year.

- It is the leading cause of death among women aged 35–49.
- The highest number of deaths occur in the 75–79 age group.

These statistics are frightening, but relatively simple changes to your diet and lifestyle can help to reduce your risk. Early detection and treatment also mean the disease is often curable.

What Is Breast Cancer?

Breast cancer develops when a single breast cell escapes from the mechanisms controlling its normal growth and development. Rather than dividing occasionally to replace old, worn-out breast cells, it continues to divide repeatedly, producing more and more abnormal 'daughter' cells. In many cases, the immune system recognizes these cells as dangerous and rapidly destroys them. If this fails, however, the abnormal cells continue to divide and invade surrounding tissues. Eventually, a detectable lump (tumour) develops, which is not usually painful in the early stages. Once the tumour has reached a certain size, a few abnormal cells may break away and spread through blood and lymph vessels to other parts of the body, where they take root and continue growing. This process is known as *metastasis* and can form so-called *secondaries* (metastases) in nearby lymph glands, bones, the lungs, brain or liver. Once breast cancer spreads like this, it is much more difficult to treat. That's why early detection of breast lumps is so important.

How Does It Develop?

Researchers are still unsure exactly how breast cancer develops. There are several different forms of the disease, which are told apart by the appearance of the cells under a microscope. Different cancers are probably triggered by different factors in different women. Possibilities include:

- the switching-on of an inherited, previously inactive (latent) gene that increases the risk of breast cancer
- damage to the genetic material from environmental pollution, free radicals (harmful by-products of metabolism) or a virus.

Who Gets It?

Breast cancer seems to run in families. It is now believed that 1 in 5 cases is linked to family history – twice as many as previously thought. For example:

- If you have no close relatives (mother, sister, daughter) with the disease, your risk of breast cancer is lower than average, at 1 in 14.
- If your mother was diagnosed with breast cancer over the age of 50, your risk is estimated as 1 in 6.
- If your mother was diagnosed with breast cancer under the age of 50, your risk of the disease could be as high as 1 in 4.
- If breast cancer has affected several generations in your family, your risk could be as high as 1 in 2.

The most likely cause of this increased risk is through inheriting a breast cancer gene. One gene in particular, called BRCA1 (on chromosome 17), is thought to be responsible for at least half of all cases. Other women who may be at increased risk of breast cancer include those who:

- started their periods aged 12 or younger
- have not had children
- have their first child after the age of 30
- have not breastfed
- have a late menopause
- use HRT for longer than 10 years (counting from the age of 50)

These factors all increase a woman's lifetime exposure to the female hormone, oestrogen. Many breast tumour cells contain oestrogen receptors which seem to stimulate tumour growth, although not all breast cancers are hormone-dependent.

Other factors that have been linked with an increased risk of breast cancer include obesity, drinking excessive amounts of alcohol, smoking cigarettes and eating a diet that is high in fat (especially animal fat) and low in fruit, vegetables and fibre.

Breast Cancer and HRT

A 50-year-old woman not on HRT has an 8 per cent risk of developing breast cancer and a 3 per cent chance of dying from it. Some studies suggest that using HRT for more than 10 years increases the risk of developing the disease from 8 to 10 per cent, though it does not increase the risk of dying from it. This is because women taking HRT receive excellent health screening, and breast lumps are picked up at an early, treatable stage.

A more recent trial found that of over 1,000 women aged 50–64 who had taken HRT for 8 years, there was no overall association between the risk of breast cancer and having taken HRT.

More importantly, research shows that, among women who had taken HRT for at least 15 years following previous breast cancer therapy, there was no increased risk of a recurrence of the disease even in those whose tumours were oestrogen-sensitive. This suggests that, as many doctors now believe, a history of breast cancer is no longer an absolute contraindication to taking HRT.

Most doctors are happy to prescribe HRT for 5–10 years (counting from the age of 50) before advising that you stop treatment. This gives maximum benefit against CHD and osteoporosis while minimizing any additional risk of developing breast cancer. Some women with an increased risk of breast cancer (such as a strong family history) may be advised – and understandably prefer – not to take it, however.

Early Detection

Ninety per cent of breast lumps are found by women or their partners. It is important to check your own breasts regularly. Aim to be breast aware and to know how your own breasts feel. Some breasts are naturally more lumpy than others, but subtle changes can be detected. Try to check your breasts at least once a month – after your period if you are still menstruating, otherwise aim for an easily remembered date such as the first of each month.

- Look at your breasts in a mirror, and check for any changes in size, shape or colour. Inspect your reflection with your arms by your sides, lifted into the air, and then with your hands pressed firmly into your hips – this helps to show up puckering, dimpling or a lump.
- Check your nipples for any change such as suddenly turning inwards, or any discharge.
- Next, lie back (in the bath or on a bed) and examine one breast at a time. Raise an arm and rest it behind your head – then check the breast on that side with your other hand. Use the flat of your first three fingers (not your fingertips) and use small, firm, circular movements, making sure you feel under your nipple, too. Then bring the raised arm down by your side and continue feeling the same breast up as far as your collar-bone and out into your armpit. Repeat on the other side. If you are unsure about how to go about examining yourself in this way, ask your practice nurse to show you how.

Women aged 50–65 years will be offered screening mammography on a regular basis. This x-ray test can pick up breast cancer changes 2 years earlier, on average, than self-examination alone. Women under this age who have a strong family history of breast cancer may be offered screening mammography too. Ask your doctor for details.

What to Do If You Find a Lump

One in three women will discover a lump in her breast at some time during her life. The important thing is not to panic. Nine out of ten breast lumps are benign fibrous lumps (fibroadenomas – also known as *breast mice*) or fluid-filled cysts, but all need to be investigated just in case. It is not easy for a doctor to tell between a lump that is cancerous and one that is not, especially in the early stages. A biopsy to remove cells and examine them under a microscope is the safest option. If you find a lump, tell your doctor straightaway – your GP would much rather see you, even if nothing is wrong, than have you neglect a potentially serious condition.

Early Diagnosis

Most lumps are investigated by a procedure known as needle aspiration – a fine needle is inserted under local anaesthetic (though this is not always necessary) and a few cells collected using a syringe. Occasionally, you may be advised to have the lump removed under a local or general anaesthetic instead. The cells are then examined under a microscope to detect cancerous changes.

Even if the results show that you do have breast cancer, try to think positive. Early diagnosis and treatment often result in a cure. A 10-year study has found that self-examination cuts breast cancer deaths by 20 per cent, as more cancers are detected at a non-invasive stage.

The care of women with breast lumps and breast cancer is undergoing a revolution. Ideally, the minimum standard of care every woman with a breast lump should expect includes:

- prompt referral by a GP to a team specializing in the diagnosis and treatment of breast cancer
- a firm diagnosis within 4 weeks of referral
- the opportunity for a confirmed diagnosis before consenting to treatment, including surgery
- access to a specialist breast care nurse trained to provide practical and emotional support
- full information about types of surgery (including breast reconstruction where appropriate) and the role of medical treatment (such as radiotherapy, chemotherapy, drugs, etc.)
- a full explanation about the aims and benefits of treatment and possible side-effects
- as much time as needed to consider treatment options
- a sensitive and complete breast prosthesis fitting service, where appropriate
- the opportunity to meet a former breast cancer patient who has been trained to offer support
- information on support services available to patients and their families.

Treatment Options

Breast cancer is not a death sentence – improvements in detection and treatment mean that of the 26,000 women who develop breast cancer in the UK each year, 62 per cent survive for at least 5 years and, of these, over 40 per cent survive long term.

If you are diagnosed as having breast cancer you are likely to have some form of surgery. Your cancer specialist needs to advise you whether removal of the lump alone is sufficient, or whether a mastectomy is your best option for a cure. The next decision is whether you would then benefit from radiotherapy, chemotherapy and/or an anti-oestrogen drug called tamoxifen which encourages hormone-sensitive breast tumours to shrink. When advising you about these decisions, the specialist needs to weigh up several factors, including:

- the size of the tumour
- the type of cells it contains
- how aggressive they are
- what stage your disease has reached.

Breast cancer is staged as follows:

Stage 1   small, movable tumour confined to the breast
Stage 2   as Stage 1, but with spread to local lymph nodes
Stage 3   locally advanced tumour, possibly attached to
           chest muscles
Stage 4   spread elsewhere in the body.

For women whose breast cancer is discovered while it is still small and in the early stages (1 or 2), world-wide research shows reassuringly that removal of the lump plus a course of radiotherapy is as safe and effective as removal of the whole breast (mastectomy). For both types of treatment, around 70 per cent of women are still alive 10 years later. Just as importantly, providing the cancer lump is small only 1 woman in 10 having a so-called *lumpectomy* will need further breast surgery.

What Can Be Done to Prevent It?

Diet and lifestyle are thought to be important in affecting your risk of breast cancer. The disease is rare in Japan, yet Japanese women moving to the West and changing to a typical Western diet lose this protection and are just as likely to develop breast cancer as a Western woman. The traditional Japanese diet is low in fat, especially saturated fat, and consists of rice, soy products (such as soybeans, soymeal, tofu) and fish together with grains and yellow-green vegetables. It is full of vitamins, minerals, fibre and protective plant hormones (isoflavonoids) thought to protect against certain cancers – especially of the breast in women, and of the prostate gland in men.

To decrease your risk of breast cancer, it is worth:

- following a low-fat, high-fibre diet – in particular, cut back on your intake of saturated (animal) fats
- eating 5 servings of fruit or vegetables per day – these contain the antioxidant vitamins C, E and betacarotene, which protect against both CHD and cancer
- losing any excess weight – fatty tissues can create oestrogen hormone from other circulating hormones
- taking regular exercise
- sticking to within the recommended safe maximum alcohol intake of 2–3 units per day for women (1 unit is equivalent to a 100-ml glass wine, 1 pub measure spirits or 300 ml normal strength beer).

Chapter Eight

COMPLEMENTARY THERAPIES

Many women with menopausal symptoms seek help from alternative therapists. There are many reasons for this, of which the most common is that you may not be able – or willing – to take hormone replacement therapy. When choosing an alternative practitioner, bear in mind that standards of training and experience vary widely. Where possible:

- Select a therapist on the basis of personal recommendation from a satisfied client whom you know and whose opinion you trust.
- Check what qualifications the therapist has, and check his or her standing with the relevant umbrella organization for that therapy. The organization will be able to tell you what training their members have undertaken and their code of ethics, and can refer you to qualified practitioners in your area.
- Find out how long your course of treatment will last and how much it is likely to cost.
- Ask how much experience the practitioner has had in treating menopausal symptoms, and about his or her rate of success.

The following complementary therapies have helped many women going through the menopause, but just as with orthodox medicine, not every treatment will suit every individual.

ACUPUNCTURE

Acupuncture is based on the belief that life energy (*chi* or *qi*) flows through the body along 12 different channels called meridians. When this energy flow becomes blocked, symptoms of illness are triggered. By inserting fine needles into specific acupuncture points overlying these meridians, blockages are overcome and the flow of *qi* corrected or altered to relieve symptoms. Altogether, there are 365 acupoints in the body; your therapist will select which points to use depending on your individual symptoms. Fine, disposable needles are used, which cause little if any discomfort. You may notice a slight pricking sensation, or an odd tingling buzz as the needle is inserted a few millimetres into the skin. The needles are usually left in place for up to 20 minutes, and may be twiddled periodically. Sometimes a small cone of dried herbs is ignited and burned near the active acupoint to warm the skin. This is known as moxibustion. The best known effect of *qi* manipulation is pain relief (local anaesthesia).

Research suggests that acupuncture causes the release of heroin-like chemicals in the body which act as natural painkillers. Acupuncture can be effective in treating menopausal symptoms, including emotional ones such as depression and anxiety.

Acupressure is similar to acupuncture, but instead of inserting needles at selected points along the meridians, they are stimulated using firm thumb pressure or fingertip massage. The best-known example of acupressure is Shiatsu massage. This is particularly effective if combined with aromatherapy essential oils for a therapeutic massage.

AROMATHERAPY

Aromatherapy essential oils have powerful effects on your moods – the part of the brain that detects smell messages from the nose (olfactory bulbs) is closely linked with the emotional centre in the brain (the limbic system). Oils are also absorbed from the skin into the circulation and can have powerful effects on the body. This is particularly noticeable in those oils that have diuretic properties. If you want a good demonstration of how substances added to the skin can penetrate the body, try rubbing a cut clove of garlic on the sole of your foot – within half an hour, the odour of garlic will be detectable on your breath.

Always use aromatherapy oils in a diluted form (such as adding to a carrier oil), as some neat oils can irritate tissues. Use them to massage into the skin, add to bathwater or be diffused into the air to scent your room.

Anise: can help to relieve pre-menstrual symptoms
Basil: helps to regulate irregular periods; can clear the mind
Bergamot: antidepressant; can help to relieve pre-menstrual symptoms
Birch: has diuretic properties
Black pepper: has sensual properties that can help to improve your sex drive
Cardamom: can help to relieve pre-menstrual symptoms
Cedarwood: has diuretic properties
Chamomile: antidepressant; helps to relieve hot flushes and sweating; has diuretic properties; helps to regulate irregular periods; can help painful periods
Cinnamon: helps to relieve vaginal dryness
Clary-sage: antidepressant; can help to alleviate oestrogen-withdrawal symptoms; helps to relieve hot flushes and sweating; helps to regulate irregular periods; can help to relieve pre-menstrual symptoms; helps to relieve vaginal dryness
Cypress: helps to relieve hot flushes and sweating; helps to regulate irregular periods; can help painful periods; can help to relieve pre-menstrual symptoms; helps to relieve vaginal dryness
Fennel: can help alleviate oestrogen-withdrawal symptoms; has diuretic properties; helps to regulate irregular periods; helps to relieve vaginal dryness
Geranium: antidepressant; helps to relieve hot flushes and sweating; has diuretic properties; helps to regulate irregular periods; can help to relieve pre-menstrual symptoms; helps to relieve vaginal dryness

Grapefruit: antidepressant; helps to relieve hot flushes and sweating; can help to relieve pre-menstrual symptoms; can clear the mind

Hyacinth: can help to relieve pre-menstrual symptoms; helps to relieve vaginal dryness

Hyssop: helps to regulate irregular periods

Jasmine: antidepressant; can help to relieve pre-menstrual symptoms; has sensual properties that can help to improve your sex drive

Jonquil: can help to relieve pre-menstrual symptoms

Juniper: has diuretic properties; helps to regulate irregular periods; can help painful periods

Lavender: antidepressant; helps to regulate irregular periods; can help to relieve pre-menstrual symptoms; helps to relieve vaginal dryness

Lemon: helps to relieve hot flushes and sweating; has diuretic properties

Lime: helps to relieve hot flushes and sweating

Mandarin: antidepressant; can help to relieve pre-menstrual symptoms

Marjoram: helps to regulate irregular periods

Melissa: antidepressant; helps to relieve vaginal dryness

Mimosa: antidepressant

Myrrh: helps to regulate irregular periods

Neroli: antidepressant; helps to relieve vaginal dryness; has sensual properties that can help to improve your sex drive

Nutmeg: helps to regulate irregular periods; can help painful periods; helps to relieve vaginal dryness

Orange: antidepressant

Patchouli: has sensual properties that can help to improve your sex drive

Peppermint: has diuretic properties; helps to regulate irregular periods; can help painful periods

Pimento: has sensual properties that can help to improve your sex drive

Rose: antidepressant; helps to relieve hot flushes and sweating; helps to regulate irregular periods; can help to relieve pre-menstrual symptoms

Rose maroc: has sensual properties that can help to improve your sex drive

Rosemary: helps to regulate irregular periods; can help painful periods; can clear the mind

Rose otto: has sensual properties that can help to improve your sex drive

Sage: helps to relieve hot flushes and sweating; helps to regulate irregular periods; can help painful periods; can help to relieve pre-menstrual symptoms

Sandalwood: antidepressant; helps to relieve vaginal dryness; has sensual properties that can help to improve your sex drive

Star anise: can help alleviate oestrogen-withdrawal symptoms

Tarragon: can help alleviate oestrogen-withdrawal symptoms; can help painful periods

Thyme: helps to relieve hot flushes and sweating; helps to regulate irregular periods; can clear the mind

Tuberose: has sensual properties that can help to improve your sex drive

Vetiver: has sensual properties that can help to improve your sex drive

Ylang ylang: antidepressant; helps to relieve vaginal dryness; has sensual properties that can help to improve your sex drive.

As smell and memory areas in the brain are closely linked, you can improve your learning power by imprinting a fact while smelling a particular aromatherapy scent (for example in a diffuser or on a hanky). When you want to recall this fact, you can do so more easily by sniffing the same scent again. Use a different blend of oils for each learning process, and only smell the same blend again when you need to recall a particular bit of information. As a test, try learning a shopping list when smelling a new mix of 3 or 4 oils. In the supermarket, smell the same scent on a hanky and see how well you remember the items you need. Good oils to use can be selected from the following:

Basil: for clarity
Bergamot: for extra confidence

Black pepper: to overcome emotional blocks and mental
exhaustion
Cardamom: for clarity
Coriander: for improved memory
Ginger: to help overcome forgetfulness
Lemon: for better concentration
Rosemary: for improved memory.

HERBALISM

For women who are unwilling or unable to take HRT – or drugs
such as clonidine to relieve hot flushes – there are alternative
options to help relieve their symptoms. While natural herbs cannot totally replace the long-term benefits of HRT on bones or the
heart, many plants contain chemicals – including natural hormone
building-blocks – which can help to relieve some menopausal
symptoms and problems.

Phytotherapy – the use of plant extracts for healing – is one of
the most exciting areas of medical research. Traditional herbs
have provided orthodox medicine with many powerful drugs
including aspirin (from the willow tree), digoxin (from the fox-
glove) and even potent new cancer treatments such as paclitax-
el (from the Pacific Yew tree). World-wide, specialists known
as ethnobiologists are continually seeking new products from
among the traditional herbs used by native healers. The Ama-
zon has proved to be one of the richest sources, providing a
wide range of traditional remedies.

Different parts of different plants are used – roots, stems, flow-
ers, leaves, bark, sap, fruit or seeds – depending on which has the
highest concentration of active ingredient. In most cases these
materials are dried and ground to produce a powder which is
made into a tea, or packed into capsules for easy swallowing.

The following herbs all have medicinal uses to help ease
menopausal symptoms. Doses vary depending on whether
you are using dried preparations, tinctures or extracts in the
form of tablets or capsules. Always follow the dosage instruc-
tions on the packet.

It is also possible to make up your own infusions from fresh or dried herbs you collect yourself. Several good books are available to guide you on this, such as *The Herb Society's Complete Medicinal Herbal* by Penelope Ody (Dorling Kindersley) and *The Encyclopedia of Medicinal Plants* by Andrew Chevallier (Dorling Kindersley).

Black Cohosh (Cimicifuga racemosa)

The dried root of Black Cohosh is used as a relaxant and a uterine stimulant to treat many gynaecological symptoms such as:

- painful periods
- irregular periods
- delayed menstruation
- uterine cramps, including labour pains
- sex hormone imbalances
- pre-menstrual syndrome.

It contains oestrogen-like plant hormones and therefore helps to overcome menopausal symptoms due to oestrogen withdrawal.

Black Cohosh also has sedative and anti-inflammatory actions, helping to treat rheumatoid arthritis, osteo-arthritis, myalgia (muscle pain) and neuralgia (nerve pain).

As Black Cohosh stimulates the womb, it should not be taken during pregnancy.

Blackcurrant Leaves (Ribes nigrum)

Blackcurrant leaves contain chemicals which help to overcome hot flushes and night sweats during the menopause. It is also used traditionally to reduce fevers, help fluid retention, boost appetite and to relieve rheumatic pains.

Chaste Berry (Vitex agnus-castus)

The ripe berries of the Chaste Tree stimulate the pituitary gland and normalize its function. This means that if too much of a particular hormone is being produced, Chaste Berry damps down secretion, while if not enough is being made, it boosts production. Research suggests that the Chaste Berry contains chemicals which inhibit the release of Follicle Stimulating Hormone (FSH) in the brain and increase production of Leutinizing Hormone (LH). As many menopausal symptoms – especially hot flushes and night sweats – have been linked with high levels of FSH, Chaste Berry is often very helpful at this time of life. It increases progesterone activity in the body and is also used to help:

- painful periods
- pre-menstrual syndrome
- mood swings
- hormone balance after stopping the oral contraceptive Pill
- breastfeeding
- post-natal depression.

Cranberry

If you are prone to recurrent urinary symptoms, especially cystitis, you may be helped by drinking cranberry juice. New research shows that people drinking 300 ml of cranberry juice a day are almost half (42 per cent) as likely to develop pus cells in the urine than those not drinking it. Furthermore, if pus cells do appear in the urine, the odds of these still being present 1 month later are only a quarter of those in people not drinking cranberry juice.

Dandelion (Taraxacum officinalis)

Dandelion is one of the most widely used herbal remedies. It stimulates removal of toxins from the body and is a powerful diuretic as well as being a rich source of potassium. It helps to flush excess sodium salts and fluid through the kidneys – in Mediaeval times the weed was known as 'piss-a-bed'. It is a useful treatment for the fluid retention that can occur with premenstrual bloating around the time of the menopause and may also help to reduce the unpleasant effects of night sweats. Interestingly, Dandelion does not seem to have a diuretic action in those with a normal, healthy fluid balance. Dandelion is also used:

- to stimulate the flow of bile
- to boost the metabolic rate
- to aid digestion
- as a laxative
- as a tonic
- to relieve rheumatic pains.

Dong Quai (Angelica sinensis)

Angelica root – known as Dong Quai or sometimes Dang Gui – is a traditional Chinese herb. It is used:

- as a nourishing blood tonic and for anaemia
- to stimulate the circulation
- as a laxative
- to relieve period pains
- for irregular periods.

False Unicorn (Chamaelirium luteum)

The root of the False Unicorn herb is a powerful stimulant and normalizer of the female reproductive system. It contains important building-blocks for the female hormone, oestrogen, and helps to overcome hormonal imbalances. It is used to treat gynaecological problems such as:

- menopausal symptoms
- delayed periods
- absent periods
- irregular ovulation
- pelvic pain
- threatened miscarriage
- morning sickness (although large doses can cause nausea and vomiting)

- tiredness, backache and low mood associated with the menopause.

It is especially helpful for early symptoms of the menopause.

Garlic (Allium sativum)

Garlic is a member of the lily family. Its bulbs are divided into segments known as cloves. World-wide, each person eats an average of 1 clove garlic per day. Garlic's most important effect for post-menopausal women is its ability to reduce the risk of coronary heart disease (CHD) and stroke.

Garlic tablets also improve blood flow to the brain. Taken regularly, they may help to improve your memory and concentration, as well as reducing your risk of heart disease. You will need to take doses of 600–900 mg standardized garlic tablets per day for the best effect. Garlic products made by solvent extraction or by boiling garlic in oil are less effective than tablets made from garlic that has been freeze-dried and powdered.

As garlic promotes sweating, some women may find that it makes hot flushes and night sweats worse – while others sometimes find it helps to shorten them by speeding up the process. Garlic also has other actions – it:

- increases the flow of bile
- aids digestion
- is anti-spasmodic and helps to relieve bowel spasms and coughs
- has antibacterial, antifungal and antiviral actions.

Ginseng

Korean (or Chinese) ginseng (*Panax ginseng*) and American ginseng (*Panax quinquefolium*) are useful supplements to take when you are feeling under the weather, or suffering from a relapse of symptoms that is dragging you down. Their roots contain steroid building-blocks similar to human sex hormones which are valuable in treating many menopausal symptoms.

Siberian ginseng (*Eleutherococcus senticosus*) is a similar but unrelated root used extensively to improve stamina and strength, particularly during or after illness. It helps the body to adapt to change and physical or emotional stress, and is therefore referred to as an adaptogen. Siberian ginseng has been shown to relieve hot flushes, vaginal dryness, sweats and anxiety. It can also boost immunity – Russian research suggests that those taking it regularly have a third fewer days off work due to health problems than those not taking it.

Make sure you buy a good quality product from a reputable company – cheap versions may contain very little active ingredient. Analysis of 50 ginseng products sold in 11 countries found that 6 contained no ginseng at all, and others only 1.9 to 9 per cent ginseng by weight. Do not take ginseng if you have high blood pressure or suffer from an oestrogen-dependent condition such as some gynaecological cancers. It is best to avoid taking stimulants such as caffeine while taking ginseng.

Ginkgo (Ginkgo biloba)

The Ginkgo biloba (or Maidenhair) tree is one of the oldest known plants and is sometimes described as a living fossil – it is virtually identical to trees existing 200 million years ago. Its leaves contain unique chemicals – gingkosides – that improve blood flow throughout the body, especially the brain, hands and feet.

Ginkgo is one of the most popular health supplements in Europe. Many people find that it helps to improve their memory and concentration as well as easing dizziness and improving circulation in the limbs. Ginkgo is also used to treat:

- irregular heartbeat
- varicose veins
- haemorrhoids
- leg ulcers
- chilblains
- tinnitus
- anxiety.

Ginkgo seeds have additional astringent, antifungal and anti-bacterial actions. They are used in China to treat asthma, chesty coughs, excess mucus, urinary incontinence and urinary frequency.

Hawthorn (Crategus oxycantha and C. monogyna)

The flowering tops of the Hawthorn bush contain chemicals which help to relax peripheral blood vessels, improve circulation to the heart, reduce the risk of angina and normalize blood pressure. These effects are still being researched in the search for new drugs. For menopausal women, Hawthorn tops are useful to:

- reduce heavy menstrual bleeding
- relieve hot flushes
- discourage fluid retention by boosting the circulation
- help depression or anxiety.

It is also used to treat diarrhoea.

Horsetail (Equisetum arvense)

Horsetail is an ancient plant related to trees growing on the earth 270 million years ago. It has brittle, jointed stems which, when dried, make a mildly diuretic remedy that can help to reduce pre-menstrual bloating associated with menopausal symptoms. Horsetail also tones the urinary tract and can help to reduce the embarrassing effects of stress incontinence, as well as reducing fluid retention. One of its most useful actions for menopausal women is that it stops excessive sweating and is therefore a useful treatment for hot flushes and night sweats. It is also used to:

- staunch bleeding and hasten wound healing
- reduce blood loss in heavy periods
- improve the circulation
- treat skin conditions
- increase urinary flow and reduce urinary infection
- control bedwetting
- improve prostate function in men.

Motherwort (Leonurus cardiaca)

The leaves of Motherwort have been used since Roman times to ease palpitations, regulate a fast pulse and lower blood pressure. It is effective in relieving anxiety and nervous tension around the time of the menopause; it also has several other gynaecological uses, including:

- stimulating menstrual flow
- easing period pains
- bringing on a late period which has been delayed by emotional shock
- infertility
- hot flushes.

As it is a uterine stimulant, it is not usually advised during pregnancy (with the exception of labour).

Oats (Avena sativa)

Oat seeds are used as a tonic for the nervous system, especially when you are exhausted or feeling low, depressed or under stress. It is a useful source of B group vitamins, which are also needed in extra amounts during times of stress such as the menopause. As the entire plant (known as Oatstraw) contains plant hormone building-blocks, it is also used as a general aid for women suffering from oestrogen- or thyroid-deficiency. Oatbran has been shown to help reduce high blood cholesterol levels and, taken regularly, can ease constipation.

If you suffer from gluten sensitivity (coeliac disease), oats can be used with care as long as you allow the infusion or tincture to settle and just use the decanted, clear liquid.

Pfaffia

The golden root of *Pfaffia paniculata* is often referred to as the Brazilian ginseng, although it is unrelated to the Oriental varieties. Like the ginsengs, however, Pfaffia is a powerful 'adaptogen', which means it helps the body's immune system to adapt to various stresses including overwork, illness and fatigue. It is regarded as a panacea for all ills, as well as a sustaining food by local Brazilian Indians, who call it *para todo* – 'for everything'. It is a rich source of vitamins, minerals, amino acids and plant hormones which act as building-blocks for the female hormone, oestrogen. It is therefore useful for treating gynaecological problems linked with hormonal imbalances such as pre-menstrual syndrome and menopausal symptoms. Because of its hormone content, pfaffia should not be taken by pregnant women. Pfaffia is used to:

- boost energy levels
- improve physical and mental stamina
- increase concentration
- speed convalescence
- improve cellulite
- relieve pre-menstrual syndrome
- relieve menopausal symptoms
- help symptoms related to the oral contraceptive Pill
- relieve impotence
- relieve arthritis
- help maintain normal blood sugar levels in people with diabetes (use with medical supervision only).

Pfaffia can be difficult to get hold of – one source is the importers, Rio Trading (tel. 01273 570987).

Sage (*Salvia officinalis*)

Sage leaves – especially those from the Red Sage – are traditionally associated with a long, healthy life. The leaves – especially those from the purple-tinged varieties – contain chemicals which can help to reduce excessive sweating and are useful for treating menopausal hot flushes and night sweats. Try taking a bed-time drink made from honey, hot water and 3 drops of essential oil of Sage to reduce night sweats.

Sage leaves are also used traditionally to:

- reduce the flow of breastmilk
- reduce excessive salivation and perspiration

- soothe inflammation of the mouth, gums, throat and tongue
- soothe intestinal infections such as diarrhoea and vomiting
- help respiratory infections such as laryngitis and tonsillitis
- relieve indigestion (dyspepsia)
- promote wound healing (when used as a compress)
- boost memory and concentration in the elderly.

As Sage stimulates uterine contractions, it should be avoided during pregnancy – small amounts are safe for use in cooking. It should also be avoided by those with epilepsy.

Sarsaparilla (*Smilax regelii*)

Sarsaparilla contains substances that boost the action of testosterone in the body. It may be helpful in overcoming a reduced sex drive in women experiencing menopausal symptoms. It is also used to treat cystitis, psoriasis and other skin disorders and, in men, impotence and infertility. It is best avoided by women with a tendency towards excessive unwanted hair.

St John's Wort (*Hypericum perforatum*)

St John's Wort is useful around the time of the menopause to help painful periods, as a mild diuretic and to boost low mood. It has been used to treat mild depression for many years in Europe. In Germany, over 16 million people have taken the prescription version of this supplement. Research involving over 5,000 patients shows that extracts of the herb can lift mild depression within 2 weeks of starting a course of treatment – the optimum effect is reached within 6 weeks. The standardized extracts contain active ingredients known as hypericins, plus nutrients such as antioxidant bioflavonoids and vitamin C. It works at the root cause of mild depression to boost production of brain chemicals (neurotransmitters) and return your mood to its natural, even keel. Trials show it can lift low mood and improve alertness and concentration. It also helps to get rid of negative emotions such as anxiety, agitation, disinterest, insomnia, headache and despair, especially around the time of the menopause.

Wild Yam (*Dioscorea villosa*)

The dried root of the Mexican Wild Yam is famous as the original source of raw plant hormones – similar to progesterone – used in the production of the oral contraceptive Pill. It increases natural production of female hormones and is used to help a number of gynaecological problems, including:

- infertility
- morning sickness
- painful periods
- pelvic pain
- ovulation pain (mittelschmertz)
- poor milk production
- menopausal symptoms
- urinary disorders.

Wild Yam is also known as the colic root, as it relaxes smooth muscle spasm and is used to relieve:

- intestinal colic
- gallbladder spasm (bilious colic)
- diverticular pain
- rheumatoid arthritis.

Should not be taken in pregnancy except under medical supervision.

Witch Hazel (*Hamamelis virginiana*)

The leaves and bark of young Witch Hazel stems can constrict superficial blood vessels, which is why it is a popular topical remedy for cuts and grazes. Witch Hazel extracts can also be taken to reduce flushing and sweating and relieve other problems which may occur around the time of the menopause, including:

- varicose veins
- haemorrhoids
- pelvic pain due to congestion

- broken capillaries (telangiectasia) on the face
- diarrhoea.

HOMOEOPATHY

Homoeopathic medicine is based on the belief that natural substances can boost the body's own healing powers to relieve the symptoms and signs of illness. Natural substances are selected which, if used full-strength in a healthy person, would produce symptoms of the illness it is designed to treat. This is the first principle of homoeopathy: 'Like cures Like.'

The second major principle of homoeopathy is that increasing the dilution of a solution has the opposite effect, that is, increases its potency ('Less Cures More'). By diluting noxious and even poisonous substances many millions of times, their healing properties are enhanced while their undesirable side-effects are lost.

On the centesimal scale, dilutions of 100^{-6} (1 drop tincture mixed with 99 drops alcohol or water and shaken; this is then done a further 6 times, each time 1 drop of the dilution being added to 99 drops of alcohol or water) are described as potencies of 6C, dilutions of 100^{-30} are written as a potency of 30C, etc. To illustrate just how diluted these substances are, a dilution of 12C (100^{-12}) is comparable to a pinch of salt dissolved in the same amount of water as is found in the Atlantic Ocean!

Homoeopathy is thought to work in a dynamic way, boosting your body's own healing powers. The principles behind homoeopathy may be difficult to accept, yet convincing trials have shown that homoeopathic therapy is significantly better than placebos in treating many chronic (long-term) conditions including hayfever, asthma and rheumatoid arthritis.

Homoeopathic remedies should ideally be taken on their own, at least 30 minutes either before or after eating or drinking. Tablets should not be handled – tip them into the lid of the container, or onto a teaspoon to transfer them into your mouth. Then suck or chew them, don't swallow them whole.

Homoeopathic treatments are prescribed according to your

symptoms rather than any particular disease, so two women with menopausal problems will usually need different homoeopathic remedies.

Homoeopathic remedies may be prescribed by a medically-trained homoeopathic doctor on a normal NHS prescription form and dispensed by homoeopathic pharmacists for the usual prescription charge or exemption. Alternatively, you can consult a private homoeopathic practitioner or buy remedies direct from the pharmacist.

Although it is best to see a trained homoeopath who can assess your constitutional type, personality, lifestyle, family background, likes and dislikes as well as your symptoms before deciding which treatment is right for you, you may find the remedies listed below helpful.

After taking the remedies for the time stated, if there is no obvious improvement consult a practitioner. Don't be surprised if your symptoms initially get worse before they get better – persevere through this common reaction to treatment – it is a good sign which shows the remedy is working.

Period Problems

■ homoeopathic remedies that may help irregular periods: *Pulsatilla 30C* – for women with fair-hair and complexion; *Sepia 30C* – for brunettes with dark skin; *Aconite 30C* – especially if periods stop suddenly due to emotional shock; *Ignatia 30C* – especially if periods stop as a result of bereavement (take every 12 hours for up to 2 weeks).

■ homoeopathic remedies that may help heavy periods: Calc carb 30C – especially if linked with marked pre-menstrual weight gain; Sepia 30C – especially if feeling faint, dizzy or irritable (every 8 hours for up to 10 doses).

■ homoeopathic remedies that may help painful periods: Pulsatilla 30C – especially if feeling weepy; Sepia 30C – especially if symptoms include cramping pains and indifference to loved ones; Kali carb 30C – especially if associated with severe backache (hourly for up to 10 doses).

- homoeopathic remedies that may help PMS: *Sepia 30C* – especially if accompanied by lack of interest; *Calc carb 30C* – especially if linked with fluid retention; *Pulsatilla 30C* – especially if linked with depression (every 12 hours for up to 6 doses, starting the day before symptoms are expected).

Physical Menopausal Symptoms

- homoeopathic remedies that may help hot flushes: *Glonoin. 30C* (every 5 minutes until flush recedes, for up to 10 doses); *Lachesis 30C* (twice a day for up to a week).
- homoeopathic remedies that may help night sweats: *Sepia 6C* – For profuse night sweats (hourly for up to 10 doses).
- homoeopathic remedies that may help fluid retention: *Apis 30C* – especially if linked with restlessness and burning hot flushes (every hour for up to 10 doses; avoid if you may be pregnant); *Bryonia 6C* – especially if accompanied by painful breasts (every 4 hours for up to 5 days).
- homoeopathic remedies that may help vaginal dryness: *Bryonia 6C* – especially if sore and uncomfortable on movement; *Lycopodium 30C* – especially if linked with hot flushes (hourly as necessary, for up to 1 week).
- homoeopathic remedies that may help loss of sex drive: *Sepia 30C* – especially if loss of interest is severe and linked with exhaustion; *Agnus castus 30C* – especially if accompanied by general lowering of energy (every 12 hours for up to 1 week).
- homoeopathic remedies that may help urinary flow problems: *Sepia 30C* – especially if linked with dragging sensations and difficulty passing water; *Causticum 30C* – especially for stress incontinence; *Natrum mur 30C* – especially if stress incontinence is linked with vaginal dryness (4 times a day for up to 3 weeks).
- homoeopathic remedies that may help cystitis: *Cantharis 30C* – especially if you have sudden onset of urinary frequency and burning; *Staphysagria 30C* – especially if burning is severe and urine is concentrated; *Phosphorus 30C* – especially if burning continues after urination (every 30 minutes for up to 10 doses – seek medical advice if no improvement).

Emotional Menopausal Symptoms

- homoeopathic remedies that may help anxiety: *Calc carb 30C* – especially if linked with panic attacks; *Lachesis 30C* – especially if talking too much through nervousness; *Phosphorus 30C* – especially for constant underlying anxiety (every 12 hours for up to 2 weeks).
- homoeopathic remedies that may help low mood: *Pulsatilla 30C* – especially if you can't stop crying; *Ignatia 30C* – especially if your moods fluctuate wildly; *Staphysagria 30C* – especially if sadness is tinged with anger; *Nux vomica 30C* – especially if linked with irritability, overwork and stress; *Arsen. alb 30C* – especially if linked with feelings of restlessness (every 12 hours for up to 2 weeks).
- homoeopathic remedies that may help insomnia: *Coffea 30C* – especially if you can't relax; *Nux vomica 30C* – especially if lack of sleep has made you irritable; *Aconite 30C* – especially if sleeplessness is linked with anxiety (1 hour before going to bed and repeat if you wake up or can't get to sleep).

Bach Rescue Remedy

This homoeopathic preparation is designed to help you cope with life's ups and downs and reduce the physical and emotional symptoms of stress and chronic illness. It contains 5 flower essences: Cherry Plum, Clematis, Impatiens, Rock Rose and Star of Bethlehem, preserved in brandy. Add 4 drops of Rescue Remedy to a glass of water and sip slowly, every 3 to 5 minutes, holding the liquid in your mouth for a while before you swallow. Alternatively, place 4 drops directly under your tongue. Useful for acute recurrences of symptoms that leave you feeling unable to cope.

After completing a course of homoeopathy, you will usually feel much better in yourself with a greatly improved sense of well-being that helps you to cope with any remaining symptoms in a much more positive way.

REFLEXOLOGY

This technique was used in China over 5,000 years ago and was also popular with the ancient Egyptians. Reflexology is based on the principle that points in the feet – known as reflexes – are directly related to other parts of the body. Massage over these reflexes can detect areas of tenderness and subtle textural changes which help to pinpoint problems in various organs, including the gut. By working on these tender spots with tiny pressure movements, nerves are thought to be stimulated that pass messages to distant organs, to relieve symptoms. Some people going through the menopause have found reflexology helpful.

Chapter Nine

LIFESTYLE AND DIETARY CHANGES

Diet and lifestyle are so important to hormone balance that relatively simple changes such as stopping smoking and improving nutrition can delay the menopause by as much as 3 or 4 years. Nutritional changes can also reduce the number of menopausal symptoms you experience, as well as helping you avoid middle-age spread.

There are three main ways in which your diet and nutritional state affects your hormone balance:

1. through the types of fat and fibre you eat
2. the natural plant hormones (phytoestrogens) present in your food
3. the amount of vitamins, minerals and trace elements you obtain.

Researchers have found that a high-fat, low-fibre diet is associated with relatively high levels of circulating oestrogen. As a result, people following this type of eating pattern are more likely to develop hormone-dependent cancers such as those of the breast or prostate gland. Red meat is the food with the strongest positive link to advanced breast or prostate cancer, while there seems to be no link between intake of dairy products – except possibly butter. Women who have followed a lifelong high-fat, low-fibre diet are more likely to have menopausal symptoms of oestrogen withdrawal – their tissues are used to a relatively high level of circulating hormones, and they seem to tolerate the menopausal drop less well.

However, switching to a healthier, low-fat, high-fibre diet around the time of the menopause can also make symptoms of oestrogen withdrawal worse (by lowering your oestrogen levels further), unless you follow a Japanese-style diet full of protective, natural plant hormones. These can damp down menopausal symptoms yet at the same time protect against cancer of the breast (or of the prostate gland in men) by stimulating production of a protein (SHBG – sex hormone binding globulin) that mops up free circulating oestrogen in the blood so that it is transported more efficiently around the body and smoothes out hormone fluctuations and imbalances.

The traditional Japanese diet is low in fat, especially saturated fat, and consists of rice, soy products (such as soybeans, soymeal, tofu) and fish together with legumes, grains and yellow-green vegetables such as cruciferous plants – these include exotic members of the cabbage and turnip families (kohlrabi; Chinese leaves). Soy and cruciferous plants are a rich source of isoflavonoids – weak plant oestrogens (phytoestrogens) which are converted into biologically active hormone-like substances by intestinal bacteria. Many vegetables contain natural oestrogen-like plant hormones known as phytoestrogens, including:

soya beans and soy products
green and yellow vegetables
broccoli
celery
fennel
liquorice
rhubarb
linseed
ginseng.

Eating too much fibre can actually make your menopausal symptoms worse, however. A large percentage of hormones excreted from the liver into the bile and then into the gut are usually reabsorbed into the circulation again before being voided. If you eat too much fibre, this can bind some of the oestrogen and increase the amount cleared from the body. Unless you have problems with constipation, it is a good idea not to increase your intake of fibre suddenly at this time of life, but to increase it slowly up to recommended levels of around 30 g per day.

ESSENTIAL FATTY ACIDS

Evening Primrose Oil (EPO) is a rich source of an essential fatty acid called GLA (gamma linolenic acid – sometimes shortened to gamolenic acid). This is a vital building-block for hormones and hormone-like substances called prostaglandins which are also involved in inflammation, blood clotting and immunity.

While some GLA can be made in the body from other dietary essential fatty acids, this reaction is easily blocked by a number of factors, including:

- eating too much saturated (animal) fat
- eating too many trans-fatty acids (such as found in margarines)
- eating too much sugar
- drinking too much alcohol
- deficiency of vitamins and minerals, especially vitamin B_6, zinc and magnesium
- increasing age
- crash dieting
- smoking cigarettes
- exposure to pollution.

When you do not get adequate amounts of essential fatty acids from your diet, your metabolism can make do with the next best fatty acids available (such as those derived from saturated fats), but as a result prostaglandin and hormone imbalances are common. This can increase your risk of developing inflammatory diseases, cyclical breast pain, irregular periods, menopausal symptoms, blood clots and dry, itchy skin. Evening Primrose Oil can naturally smooth out these problems – it is so effective that some doctors prescribe it to treat eczema and mastalgia (breast pain).

The action of GLA is boosted by vitamin E, which helps to preserve it in the body. It is therefore important to take a supplement containing both GLA and vitamin E, or to take vitamin E capsules at the same time.

Certain vitamins and minerals are also needed during the metabolism of essential fatty acids. These are vitamin C, vitamin B_6, vitamin B_3 (niacin), zinc and magnesium. If you are taking Evening Primrose Oil you should therefore ensure that your intake of these is adequate (such as by taking a multinutrient supplement).

The only people who should not take EPO are those who are allergic to it and those with a particular rare nervous disorder known as temporal lobe epilepsy. Check with your doctor.

VITAMINS AND MINERALS

It is estimated that only 1 in 10 people get all the necessary vitamins and minerals from diet alone. These are needed for:

- burning fuel for energy
- healthy cell membranes, skin and bones
- the production and action of hormones and enzymes
- fighting infections
- proper healing.

Even if only one nutrient is in short supply, it can affect your metabolism, immune system and hormone balance, which may be enough to tip the scales and make your menopausal symptoms worse. If taking a vitamin and mineral supplement, for example, it's best to take one supplying around 100 per cent of the recommended daily amount (RDA) of as many vitamins and minerals as possible.

The recommended vitamin and mineral intake that will supply the needs of the majority of the population are:

VITAMIN	RDA
Vitamin A (retinol)	800 mcg
Vitamin B_1 (thiamin)	1.4 mg
Vitamin B_2 (riboflavin)	1.6 mg
Vitamin B_3 (niacin)	18 mg
Vitamin B_5 (pantothenic acid)	6 mg

Vitamin B$_6$ (pyridoxine)	2 mg
Vitamin B$_{12}$ (cyanocobalamin)	1 mcg
Biotin	0.15 mg
Folic Acid	200 mcg
Vitamin C	60 mg
Vitamin D	5 mcg
Vitamin E	10 mg

MINERAL

Calcium	800 mg–1,500 mg
Iodine	150 mcg
Iron	14 mg
Magnesium	300 mg
Phosphorus	800 mg
Zinc	15 mg

Minor vitamin and mineral deficiencies are common. Lack of nutrients is rarely severe enough to cause the sort of deficiency diseases seen in the third world (such as scurvy, beri-beri), but they can be enough to affect your immunity and hormone balance and to increase your risk of a number of health problems:

- 60 per cent of the population do not obtain the new EC recommended daily amounts (RDA) of 60 mg vitamin C on a regular basis.
- 90 per cent of the population do not obtain the recommended 10 mg vitamin E.
- 99 per cent of people obtain less than 2 mg betacarotene per day from their food – there is no separate RDA for betacarotene, but the National Cancer Institute in the US suggests a minimum intake of 6 mg betacarotene per day (equivalent to 100 ml carrot juice) to protect against cancer.
- average intakes of vitamin B$_1$ and B$_2$ are below recommended levels
- 50 per cent of adults obtain less vitamin B$_6$ than they should.

The situation with minerals is even worse. The 1993 UK Government Food Survey shows that a large proportion of the population is at risk of gross deficiency in 8 out of 13 vitamins and minerals. Compared with the new EC RDAs, the average adult only obtains:

- 53 per cent of the RDA for zinc
- 56 per cent of the RDA for vitamin D
- 68 per cent of the RDA for iron
- 78 per cent of the RDA for magnesium

and 40 per cent of people obtain less dietary calcium than recommended.

Another Government report confirms that the average intake of the mineral selenium has fallen dramatically, from 60 mcg in 1978 to just 34 mcg in 1995. The ideal intakes are 75 mcg for men and 60 mcg for women.

Even when the lowest possible intake of a mineral – the amount necessary to prevent deficiency disease – is measured, one UK Government survey found:

Proportion of Women with Intakes Below the Lower Reference Nutrient Intake

Nutrient	16–18 years LRNI %		19–50 years LRNI %		51–64 years LRNI %	
Calcium (mg)	480	27%	400	10%	400	5%
Iron (mg)	8	33%	8	26%	8	1%
Magnesium (mg)	190	39%	150	13%	150	9%
Potassium (mg)	2,000	30%	2,000	27%	2,000	23%

Dietary and Nutritional Survey of British Adults – Further Analysis MAFF. HMSO

And that's just for the lower reference nutrient intake. When you consider that optimum intakes of calcium are at least 800 mg per day (the National Osteoporosis Society would prefer that you obtained more – *see page* 79) and that menstruating women ideally need at least 14 mg iron per day, the number of women obtaining less than optimal levels of minerals is worrying.

Lack of vitamins and minerals can cause a number of common symptoms, including:

- lowered immunity
- recurrent infections
- poor wound healing
- feeling tired all the time
- mouth ulcers
- sore tongue
- cracked lips
- inflamed gums
- scaly skin
- brittle nails and hair
- pre-menstrual syndrome
- constipation
- nerve conduction problems
- muscle weakness.

To safeguard yourself against these common nutrient deficiencies, it is worth taking a good vitamin and mineral supplement to provide around 100 per cent of the RDA of as many micronutrients as possible.

DIETARY AND LIFESTYLE CHANGES TO HELP REDUCE
HOT FLUSHES

- Drink plenty of fluids, especially mineral or filtered water.
- Eat at least 5 portions of fresh fruit and vegetables per day, especially those rich in plant hormones.
- Eat more nuts and seeds.
- Eat more wholegrain cereals.
- Eat more fish – especially oily fish – or take omega-3 fish oil supplements.
- Eat little and often during the day to keep your blood sugar levels constant – fresh or dried fruit is ideal for snacks.
- Use low-fat versions of dairy products, and drink an extra pint of semi-skimmed or skimmed milk per day.

- Avoid or limit your intake of sugar, salt, tea, coffee and other caffeinated drinks.
- Avoid hot, spicy foods.
- If you smoke, try to stop.
- Avoid or limit your intake of alcohol.
- Avoid convenience, pre-processed foods and additives – eat home-made meals as often as possible.
- Reduce your salt intake.
- Take Evening Primrose Oil (1–3 g per day)
- Consider taking Siberian ginseng (*Eleutherococcus*) – doses of 400–1,200 mg per day have been shown to relieve hot flushes, vaginal dryness, sweats and anxiety. (For information on other herbs that can help – such as Sarsaparilla, St John's Wort, Dong Quai or Black Cohosh – *see pages 134-45*.)
- Consider taking a vitamin and mineral supplement as a nutritional safety net.

Tips to Help You Sleep Better If You Suffer from Night Sweats and Hot Flushes

- Try to nap during the day if you feel tired – but bear in mind that this may make sleep more difficult at night.
- Take regular exercise, as active people tend to sleep more easily.
- Avoid strenuous exercise late in the evening.
- Try to eat your evening meal before 7 p.m. and resist late-night snacks, especially of rich foods.
- Hunger is a primitive alerting response. The more hungry you are, the more difficult it is to fall asleep. Eat a healthy, wholefood diet with plenty of complex carbohydrates (such as cereals, bread, pasta) and fruit and vegetables for vitamins and minerals.
- Avoid over-indulgence in substances that interfere with sleep such as caffeine (coffee, tea, chocolate, colas) nicotine and alcohol – although alcohol may help you to fall asleep, you are likely to have a disturbed sleep once the drugged effect has worn off.
- Take time to unwind from the stresses of the day before going to bed – read a book, listen to soothing music or have a relaxing bath.

- A warm, milky drink just before going to bed will help you to relax – hot milk with cinnamon or nutmeg is better than chocolate drinks, which contain some caffeine.
- Don't drink too much fluid in the evening – a full bladder is guaranteed to disturb your rest.
- Get into the habit of going to bed at a regular time each night and getting up at the same time each morning.
- Set a bed-time routine – brushing your teeth, washing, setting the alarm clock, etc. – to set the mood for sleep.
- Make sure your bed is comfortable and your bedroom warm, dark and quiet – noise and excessive cold or heat will keep you awake. A temperature of 18–24°C is ideal.
- If you can't sleep, don't lie there tossing and turning. Get up and read or watch television for a while. If you are worried about something, write down all the things on your mind and promise yourself you will start to deal with them in the morning, when you are feeling fresher. When you feel sleepy, go back to bed and try again. If sleep does not come within 15 minutes, get up and repeat this process.
- Preserve your bedroom as a place for sleep (and sex) – don't use it for eating, working or watching television.

USEFUL ADDRESSES

AMARANT TRUST
  Grant House
  56–60 St John St
  London EC1M 4DT
  Helpline: 0171 490 1644

NATIONAL OSTEOPOROSIS SOCIETY
  PO Box 10
  Radstock
  Bath BA3 3YB
  Helpline: 01761 432472

CONTINENCE FOUNDATION
  The Dene Centre
  Castle Farm Road
  Newcastle upon Tyne
  NE3 1PH
  Helpline: 2 p.m.–7 p.m.
  Mon–Fri 0191 213 0050

ENURESIS RESOURCE AND
INFORMATION CENTRE (ERIC)
  65 St Michael's Hill
  Bristol BS2 8DZ
  Helpline: 0117 926 4920

BRITISH MIGRAINE ASSOCIATION
  178a High Road
  Byfleet
  Surrey KT14 7ED
  Helpline: 01932 352468

THE MIGRAINE TRUST
  45 Great Ormond Street
  London WC1N 3HD
  Helpline: 0171 278 2676

FURTHER READING

LIFESTYLE

Leon Chaitow, *Stress* (Thorsons)
Leonard Mervyn, *Thorsons Complete Guide to Vitamins and Minerals* (Thorsons)
Elaine Moquetter-Magee, *Eat Well for a Healthy Menopause* (Wiley)
Ariel Simkin and Judith Ayalon, *Bone Loading – Exercises for Osteoporosis* (Prion)
Felicity Smart and Dr Diana Holdright, *Heart Health for Women* (Thorsons)
Stephen Terrass, *Stress* (Thorsons)

ALTERNATIVE MEDICINE

Susan Curtis and Romy Fraser, *Natural Healing for Women* (Pandora)
David Hoffman, *The Complete Illustrated Holistic Herbal* (Element Books)
Dr Andrew Lockie and Dr Nicola Geddes, *The Complete Guide to Homeopathy* (Dorling Kindersley)
Beth MacEoin, *Homoeopathy and the Menopause* (Thorsons)
Penelope Ody, *The Herb Society's Complete Medicinal Herbal* (Dorling Kindersley)
The Reader's Digest Family Guide to Alternative Medicine
Norman Shealy (ed.), *The Complete Family Guide to Alternative Medicine* (Element Books)
Dr Melvyn Werbach, *Healing through Nutrition* (Thorsons)
Valerie Ann Worwood, *The Fragrant Pharmacy* (Bantam Books)

INDEX

aches and pains 40–41
acne 38
acupuncture 130
anxiety 42–3
aromatherapy 130–34
atherosclerosis 85–7
  see also coronary heart
    disease

bladder problems 33
breast cancer:
  early detection of 124–5
  early diagnosis of 126
  how it develops 122
  prevention 128
  the facts 121–22
  treatment options 127
  what it is 122
  who gets it 123

clitoral hood retraction 50
contraception: 57–68
  and sterilization 67–8
  barrier methods of 59–60
  hormonal methods of
    60–65
  inter uterine devices 65–7
  natural methods of 58–9
coronary heart disease 84–96

and blood cholesterol levels
  87–8
and HRT 88–9, 109–10
and syndrome X 89–90
dietary changes for health
  93–6
modifiable risk factors 91–3
risk factors 90–91
corpus luteum 8

depression *see* tearfulness and
  depression
diet and lifestyle: 150–52
  and essential fatty acids
    152–3
  vitamins and minerals
    153–6

facial hair:
  increase in 39
female reproduction:
  regulation of 10–12
food cravings 46–8

hair changes 39
heart disease *see* coronary
  heart disease
herbalism 134–45
homeopathy 145–9